Diabetes: the way towards CURE

Researched, collected and written by

Zsolt Szemerszky

First Printing: May 2016

ISBN-13: 978-1533116000

ISBN-10: 1533116008

CreateSpace Independent Publishing Platform
Amazon.com

www.zsoltszemerszky.com

Contents

Pre-words 15

Sweet Urine Disease 20

How to determine whether you have Diabetes? 27

Types of Diabetes 33

Type 1 Diabetes *37*

Type 1.5 Diabetes (LADA) *46*

Pre-Diabetes *50*

Impaired Fasting Glycaemia 51

Impaired Glucose Tolerance 53

Type 2 Diabetes *54*

Type 3 Diabetes (Alzheimer's) *61*

Gestational Diabetes *64*

The role of our Pancreas 70

What is Insulin? 73

Discovery of insulin *76*

Inhalable insulin *80*

Landmark discoveries *83*

Managing Diabetes 85

Hypoglycemia *87*

Hyperglycemia *91*

Hyperosmolar Hyperglycemic State *95*

Diabetic ketoacidosis *97*

Brittle Diabetes *102*

Measuring the blood sugar *104*

Insulin treatment *107*

Non-Invasive tools *110*

Glucose-Sensing Contact Lens 112

Diabetes tattoo 115

Measuring from the Sweat 118

Measuring on the Skin 120

Glucose Monitor Implant 123

Measuring on the Ears 124

Measuring from the Tissue fluid 126

Solutions for Parents and Relatives *129*

Possible cures 132

Pre-Diabetes *136*

Type 1 *137*

Pancreas transplantation 140

Artificial pancreas 142

Cure through Replacing Insulin-producing Cells 143

Cure through Vaccines and Immunotherapy 145

Cure through Probiotic pill 146

Type 2 *147*

Implementing the concept of “Balanced life” 148

Basic medications for Type 2 Diabetes 154

Alternative medicines 159

Marijuana 160

Protein injection 161

Surgical ways for Type 2 patients 162

Type 3 *163*

Prevention of Diabetes 165

Global burden 168

Conclusions 174

Bonus chapter: My Type 1 Diabetes story... 177

Acknowledgements 182

Liability disclaimer 186

Dedication

I dedicate this book, collection of Diabetes related information to all the fellow Diabetes sufferers and to their courageous families and relatives.

I would like to also take the chance to say a big THANK YOU to Ms Sieglinde Kratz who helped me to understand my Type 1 Diabetes when I was diagnosed with it and who showed me how to manage this life-long disease in order to have a balanced and quality life.

Furthermore I would like to also say thank you to three special persons in my life, Dodo Newman, Viviane Reziciner and Laszlo Winter, who helped me in different periods with my Diabetes.

Introduction

Zsolt Szemerszky is a National Quality Prize Winner Revenue Specialist, author, serial entrepreneur and also a fellow sufferer of Diabetes Type 1.

His aim is to help people and corporations to achieve their highest ambitions.

Being an author of multiple books, published in over 50 countries world-wide helped Zsolt Szemerszky to create business values for people and to motivate them on the road towards their aims.

One of Zsolt's most quoted sentence is:

> *"Every mountain can be climbed*
> *you just have to find the appropriate way to it.*
> *If somebody does not achieve it's goal*
> *then he/she has not done everything to achieve it.*
> *The secret of success is persistence!"*

Diabetes: the way towards CURE

Researched, collected and written by

Zsolt Szemerszky

Pre-words

"ALL TYPES OF DIABETES ARE TREATABLE."

There is a great misconception about Diabetes, but why? How is it possible that Diabetes is one of the deadliest disease which effects 8.8% of our population *(422 million people!)* and still people do not know about its seven different types. And it is a very accurate question since almost everyone knows about HIV/ AIDS which effects *"only"* 35 million people globally, which is a much lower number compared to the 422 million Diabetics.

No, **Diabetes is not about obesity.** It is much more than that. Not to mention that many people having Diabetes are not even fat. It is important that people with Diabetes, pre-Diabetes, their loved ones, employers and schools have an accurate picture of this life threatening disease.

Diabetes effects women during **pregnancy**, it effects **children** from early ages, it is the reason for men to underperform in sexual activities, it is the **5th leading cause related to death of women** and the **8th leading cause of death in overall** in people's life.

So what is Diabetes really?

A silent *(but treatable)* killer, a form of *"cancer"*. Something which definitely messes up your life and all of those who care about you. Why? Because it effects everyone starting from the pregnancy, through the young years until the elderly age. And it is definitely not just a lifestyle choice.

Just think about how could an infant choose a life-long disease when their parents are perfectly healthy?

However on the sunny side Diabetes is treatable and in 90% of the cases you have a great chance to get rid of it which sounds promising.

Medically speaking Diabetes, often referred to by doctors as Diabetes Mellitus, describes a group of metabolic diseases in which the person has high blood glucose *(blood sugar)*, either because insulin production is inadequate, or because the body's cells do not respond properly to insulin, or both.

Patients with high blood sugar will typically experience polyuria *(frequent urination)*, they will become increasingly thirsty *(polydipsia)* and hungry *(polyphagia)*.

Diabetes has seven different types and only one of them is related to your lifestyle, which is called Type 2 Diabetes.

This is the one which effects the elderly people and is mostly diagnosed with overweighted people. Also this is where we can observe that the vast majority of patients with Type 2 Diabetes initially had Pre-Diabetes. Their blood glucose levels where higher than normal, but not high enough to merit a Diabetes diagnosis. Later on the cells in the body become more and more resistant to insulin.

Studies have indicated that even at the Pre-Diabetes stage some damage to the circulatory system and the heart may already have occurred. This is also the reason why it is important to notice early the signs.

So let's see the **seven different types of Diabetes**:

➡ **Type 1**, is the juvenile Diabetes which usually effects children in a very early age, a condition where the body does not produce enough insulin.

➡ **Type 1.5**, is a form of Type 1 Diabetes that occurs in adults.

➡ **Pre-Diabetes**, when the blood glucose levels are high but not high enough for a diagnosis of Type 2 Diabetes.

➡ **Type 2**, usually effects elderly and obese people, a condition where the body produces insulin but can not use it well.

- **Type 3**, is a proposed term for Alzheimer's disease resulting in an insulin resistance in the brain.
- **Gestational Diabetes**, which affects females during the pregnancy, it is a temporary condition.
- **Diabetes Insipidus**, caused by either hormonal or kidney problems.

Interestingly from the 422 million people all around the world suffering from Diabetes almost 90% has the Type 2 Diabetes. Still, the true misconception lies in the fact that only one of the seven Diabetes types is related to your lifestyle, the Type 2 Diabetes.

All types of Diabetes are treatable. Which is a good news, however the dark side is that there is no officially announced cure yet. However while the Type 1 lasts lifetime long, the Type 2 might be treatable even without serious medications. For example there are many people who managed to get rid of their symptoms through a combination of exercise, diet and body weight control. There are other, medical ways as well such as gastric bypass surgery can reverse Type 2 Diabetes in a high proportion of patients, but this is just one of the many.

> ***Facts & Myths*** *Nr 1.*
>
> *Myth:* Diabetes is a nuisance, but not serious.
>
> *Fact:* Two thirds of Diabetes patients die prematurely from stroke or heart disease. The life expectancy of a person with Diabetes is from five to ten years shorter than that of other people. Diabetes is a serious disease.

Treatment with Diabetes is highly important because the lack of care can have serious consequences.

Diabetes can lead to complications in many parts of the body such as stroke, blindness, heart attack, kidney failure, amputations and increase the risk of dying prematurely. However people can live a long and healthy life when their Diabetes is detected and well-managed.

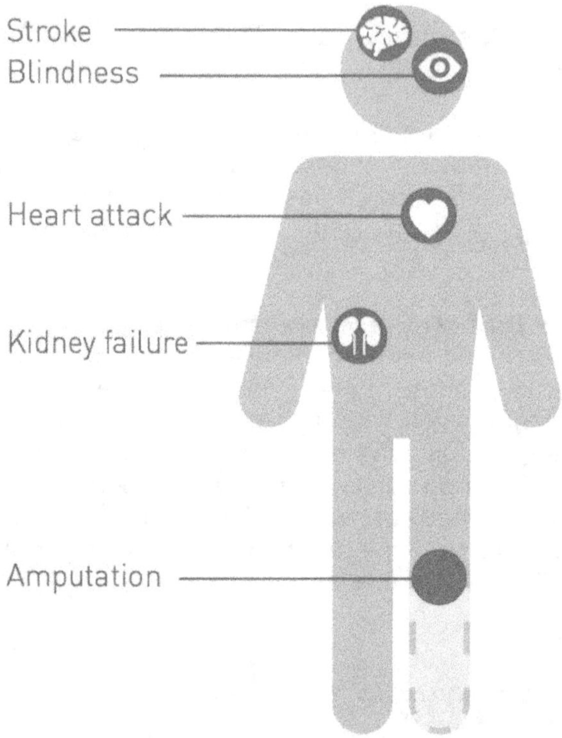

Photo credit: World Health Organization

Present book is a collection of the basic information and vocabulary of Diabetes in order to ensure you a better understanding of this disease. It will also help you to fully understand it and by this to create for yourself a better quality of life.

I am not a doctor, however I believe that being a victim also qualifies me to understand what is happening with my own body and with my fellow sufferers. So I created this book as a form of common knowledge and collection of Diabetes vocabulary.

Before you purchase this book it is good to know that **the book is also available free of charge** *(http://www.Diabetes-cure.me/*

book) since the main objective was to create an educational book reaching out to as many people as possible. So please feel free to download it and share it with as many people as possible because the ability to care for over 422 Million Diabetic people is a game changer.

Sweet Urine Disease

"IN ANCIENT CHINA PEOPLE OBSERVED THAT ANTS WOULD BE ATTRACTED TO SOME PEOPLE'S URINE, BECAUSE IT WAS SWEET."

Diabetes was one of the first diseases described with an Egyptian manuscript from c. 1500 BCE mentioning *"too great emptying of the urine"*. The first described cases are believed to be of Type 1 Diabetes.

The disease was also recognize by the ancient Greeks, Chinese, Egyptians, Indians and Persians.

The earliest surviving work with detailed reference to Diabetes is that of Aretus the Cappadocian, a Greek physician during the second century A.D.

He described patients who were passing too much water like a siphon and named the condition diabainein *(διαβαίνειν)*. The intended meaning of the word was *"excessive discharge of urine"* which is composed of δια- *(dia-)*, meaning *"through"* and βαίνειν *(bainein)*, meaning *"to go"*.

Diabetes appears to have been a death sentence in the ancient era. Hippocrates makes no mention of it, which may indicate that he felt the Diabetes disease was incurable. However Aretaeus the Cappadocian did attempt to treat it but he could not give a good prognosis and he commented that ***"life** (with Diabetes) **is short, disgusting and painful"***.

He attributed the diabainein to the moisture and coldness, reflecting the beliefs of the *"Pneumatic School"*. He hypothesized a correlation of Diabetes with other diseases and he discussed differential diagnosis from the snakebite which also provokes excessive thirst.

His work remained unknown in the West until the middle of the 16th century when in 1552, the first Latin edition was published in Venice.

Type 1 and Type 2 Diabetes were identified as separate conditions for the first time by the Indian physicians Sushruta and Charaka in 400-500 CE with Type 1 Diabetes associated with youth and Type 2 Diabetes with being overweight. Furthermore they also identified the disease and classified it as Madhumeha or *"honey urine"*.

In medieval Persia, Avicenna *(980–1037)* provided a detailed account on Diabetes Mellitus in The Canon of Medicine, *"describing the abnormal appetite and the collapse of sexual functions,"* and he documented the sweet taste of diabetic urine. Like Aretaeus before him, Avicenna recognized a primary and secondary Diabetes.

He also described diabetic gangrene and treated Diabetes using a mixture of lupine, trigonella *(fenugreek)*, and zedoary seed, which produces a considerable reduction in the excretion of sugar, a treatment which is still prescribed in modern times.

Also in the ancient China people observed that ants would be attracted to some people's urine, because it was sweet. The term *"Sweet Urine Disease"* *(táng niăo bìng (糖尿病))* was coined.

This name has also been borrowed into Korean and Japanese.

Later on around 1425, the word *"diabainein"* became *"Diabetes"* from the English adoption of the Medieval Latin Diabetes.

The word Diabetes comes from Latin diabētēs, which in turn comes from Ancient Greek διαβήτης *(diabētēs)* which literally means *"a passer through; a siphon"*.

In 1675, the British Thomas Willis added *"Mellitus"* or *"from honey"* to the term, although it is commonly referred to simply as Diabetes.

Mel in Latin means *"honey"*; the urine and blood of people with Diabetes has excess glucose, and glucose is sweet like honey.

Adding the name *"Mellitus"* was an important step to separate the Diabetes Mellitus from the Diabetes Insipidus.

They both are referred as Diabetes because they are associated with increased thirst and frequent urination. However the two are entirely separated conditions with different mechanisms.

In an everyday term Diabetes Mellitus could literally mean *"siphoning off sweet water"*.

In 1776 Matthew Dobson confirmed that the sweet taste comes from an excess of a kind of sugar in the urine and blood.

Although Diabetes has been recognized since antiquity and treatments of various efficacy have been known in various regions since the Middle Ages, and in legend for much longer, pathogenesis of Diabetes has only been understood experimentally since about 1900.

Diabetes Mellitus is classed as a metabolism disorder. Metabolism refers to the way our bodies use digested food for energy and growth.

Most of what we eat is broken down into glucose. Glucose is a form of sugar in the blood - it is the principal source of fuel for our bodies. When our food is digested, the glucose makes its way into our bloodstream. Our cells use the glucose for energy and growth.

However, glucose cannot enter our cells without insulin being present since insulin makes it possible for our cells to take in the glucose.

Insulin is a hormone that is produced by the pancreas. After eating, the pancreas automatically releases an adequate quantity of insulin to move the glucose present in our blood into the cells, as soon as glucose enters the cells blood-glucose levels drop.

A person with Diabetes has a condition in which the quantity of glucose in the blood is too elevated *(Hyperglycemia)*. This is because the body either does not produce enough insulin, or produces no insulin, or has cells that do not respond properly to the insulin the pancreas produces.

This results in too much glucose building up in the blood. Excess blood glucose eventually passes out of the body in the form of urine. So, even though the blood has plenty of glucose, the cells are not getting it for their essential energy and growth requirements.

It is incredible to state that Diabetes is one of the oldest documented disease and still, effective treatment was not developed until the early part of the 20th century, when Canadians Frederick Banting and Charles Herbert Best isolated and purified insulin in 1921 and 1922. This was followed by the development of the long-acting insulin NPH in the 1940s.

The distinction between what is now known as Type 1 Diabetes and Type 2 Diabetes was first clearly made by Sir Harold Percival *(Harry)* Himsworth, and published in January 1936. Which is just a lifetime ago.

As you can understand Diabetes is a serious, chronic disease with a lot of possible complications in many parts of the body linked to it and **it can increase the overall risk of dying prematurely**. Possible complications include heart attack, stroke, kidney failure, leg amputation, vision loss and nerve damage. In pregnancy, poorly controlled Diabetes increases the risk of fetal death and other complications.

Facts & Myths *Nr 2.*

Myth: One person can transmit Diabetes to another person.

Fact: Not true! Just like a broken leg is not infectious or contagious. A parent may pass on, through their genes to their offspring, a higher susceptibility to developing the disease.

Badly controlled Diabetes can cause:

- ➡ **Eye complications** - glaucoma, cataracts, diabetic retinopathy, and some others.
- ➡ **Neuropathy** - diabetic neuropathy is a type of nerve damage which can lead to several different problems.
- ➡ **Foot complications** - neuropathy, ulcers, and sometimes gangrene which may require that the foot be amputated.
- ➡ **Skin complications** - people with Diabetes are more susceptible to skin infections and skin disorders.
- ➡ **Heart problems** - such as ischemic heart disease, when the blood supply to the heart muscle is diminished.
- ➡ **Hypertension** - common in people with Diabetes, which can raise the risk of kidney disease, eye problems, heart attack and stroke.
- ➡ **Mental health** - uncontrolled Diabetes raises the risk of suffering from depression, anxiety and some other mental disorders.
- ➡ **Hearing loss** - Diabetes patients have a higher risk of developing hearing problems.
- ➡ **Gum disease** - there is a much higher prevalence of gum disease among Diabetes patients.
- ➡ **Gastroparesis** - the muscles of the stomach stop working properly.
- ➡ **Ketoacidosis** - a combination of ketosis and acidosis; accumulation of ketone bodies and acidity in the blood.
- ➡ **HHNS** *(Hyperosmolar Hyperglycemic Nonketotic Syndrome)* - blood glucose levels shoot up too high, and there are no ketones present in the blood or urine. It is an emergency condition.
- ➡ **Kidney disease** - uncontrolled blood pressure can lead to kidney disease.
- ➡ **PAD** *(Peripheral Arterial Disease)* - symptoms may include pain in the leg, tingling and sometimes problems walking properly.

- **Stroke** - if blood pressure, cholesterol levels, and blood glucose levels are not controlled, the risk of stroke increases significantly.
- **Erectile dysfunction** - male impotence.
- **Infections** - people with badly controlled Diabetes are much more susceptible to infections.
- **Healing of wounds** - cuts and lesions take much longer to heal.

When Diabetes is not well managed, complications develop that threaten health and endanger life. Acute complications can contribute to mortality, high medical costs and poor quality of life.

Abnormally high blood glucose can have a life-threatening impact if it triggers conditions such as Diabetic Ketoacidosis *(DKA)* in Type 1 Diabetes and Type 2 Diabetes, and Hyperosmolar coma in Type 2 Diabetes.

Abnormally low blood glucose can occur in all types of Diabetes and may result in seizures or loss of consciousness. It may happen after skipping a meal or exercising more than usual, or if the dosage of anti-diabetic medication is too high.

Over time Diabetes can damage the heart, blood vessels, eyes, kidneys and nerves, and increase the risk of heart disease and stroke.

Such damage can result in reduced blood flow, which – combined with nerve damage *(neuropathy)* in the feet – increases the chance of foot ulcers, infection and the eventual need for limb amputation.

Diabetic retinopathy is an important cause of blindness and occurs as a result of long-term accumulated damage to the small blood vessels in the retina.

Diabetes is among the leading causes of kidney failure.

Uncontrolled Diabetes **in pregnancy** can have a **devastating effect on both mother and child**, substantially increasing the risk of fetal loss, congenital malformations, stillbirth, perinatal death, obstetric complications, and maternal morbidity and mortality.

Gestational Diabetes increases the risk of some adverse outcomes for mother and offspring during pregnancy, childbirth and immediately after delivery *(pre-eclampsia and eclampsia in the mother; large for gestational age and shoulder dystocia in the offspring)*. However, it is not known what proportion of obstructed births or maternal and perinatal deaths can be attributed to Hyperglycaemia.

The combination of increasing prevalence of Diabetes and increasing lifespans in many populations with Diabetes may be leading to a changing spectrum of the types of morbidity that accompany Diabetes.

In addition to the traditional complications described above, Diabetes has been associated with increased rates of specific cancers, and increased rates of physical and cognitive disability.

This diversification of complications and increased years of life spent with Diabetes indicates a need to better monitor the quality of life of people with Diabetes and assess the impact of interventions on quality of life.

It is a sad fact that the Diabetes prevalence has doubled since 1980. Therefore Diabetes is also an important public health problem, one of four priority NonCommunicable Diseases *(NCDs)* targeted for action by world leaders. Both the number of cases and the prevalence of Diabetes have been steadily increasing over the past few decades.

In the past three decades the prevalence 1 *(age-standardized)* of Diabetes has risen substantially in countries at all income levels, mirroring the global increase in the number of people who are overweight or obese.

The global prevalence of Diabetes has grown from 4.7% in 1980 to 8.5% in 2014, during which time prevalence has increased or at best remained unchanged in every country.

The World Health Organization also raised attention in 2016 to the fact that the Eastern Mediterranean Region has experienced the greatest rise in Diabetes prevalence.

How to determine whether you have Diabetes?

"DIABETES AT LEAST DOUBLES A PERSON'S RISK OF DEATH!"

People can often have Diabetes and be completely unaware. The main reason for this is that the symptoms, when seen on their own, seem harmless. This is also the reason why Diabetes at least doubles a person's risk of death.

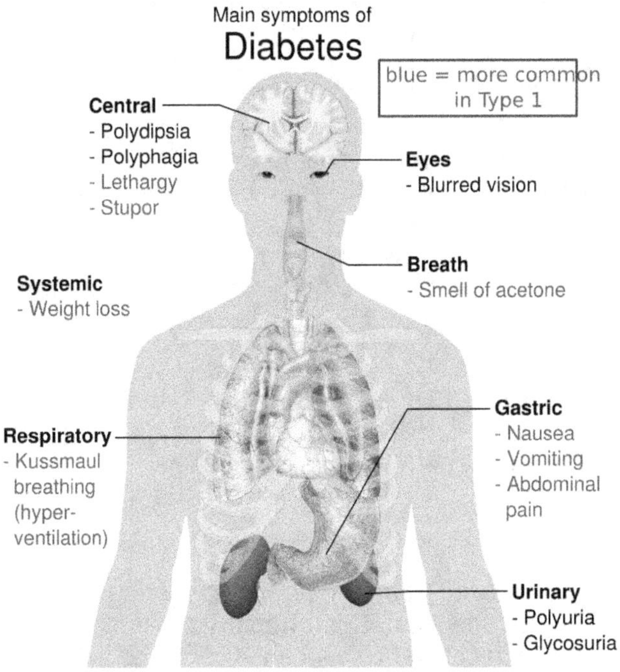

Photo credit: Mikael Häggström/WikiPedia

The earlier Diabetes is diagnosed the greater the chances are that serious complications *(which can result from having Diabetes)* can be avoided.

Here is a list of the most common Diabetes symptoms:

- **Frequent urination:** Have you been going to the bathroom to urinate more often recently? Do you notice that you spend most of the day going to the toilet? When there is too much glucose *(sugar)* in your blood you will urinate more often. If your insulin is ineffective, or not there at all, your kidneys cannot filter the glucose back into the blood. The kidneys will take water from your blood in order to dilute the glucose - which in turn fills up your bladder.
- **Disproportionate thirst:** If you are urinating more than usual, you will need to replace that lost liquid. You will be drinking more than usual. Have you been drinking more than usual lately?
- **Intense hunger:** As the insulin in your blood is not working properly, or is not there at all, and your cells are not getting their energy, your body may react by trying to find more energy - food. You will become hungry.
- **Weight gain:** This might be the result of the above symptom *(intense hunger)*.
- **Unusual weight loss:** This is more common among people with Type 1 Diabetes. As your body is not making insulin it will seek out another energy source *(the cells aren't getting glucose)*. Muscle tissue and fat will be broken down for energy. As Type 1 Diabetes is of a more sudden onset and Type 2 Diabetes is much more gradual, weight loss is more noticeable with Type 1 Diabetes.
- **Increased fatigue:** If your insulin is not working properly, or is not there at all, glucose will not be entering your cells and providing them with energy. This will make you feel tired and listless.
- **Irritability:** Irritability can be due to your lack of energy.
- **Blurred vision:** This can be caused by tissue being pulled from your eye lenses. This affects your eyes' ability to focus. With proper treatment this can be treated. There are severe cases where blindness or prolonged vision problems can occur.

- **Cuts and bruises do not heal properly or quickly:** Do you find cuts and bruises take a much longer time than usual to heal? When there is more sugar *(glucose)* in your body, its ability to heal can be undermined.
- **More skin and/or yeast infections:** When there is more sugar in your body, its ability to recover from infections is affected. Women with Diabetes find it especially difficult to recover from bladder and vaginal infections.
- **Itchy skin:** A feeling of itchiness on your skin is sometimes a symptom of Diabetes.
- **Gums are red and/or swollen - Gums pull away from teeth:** If your gums are tender, red and/or swollen this could be a sign of Diabetes. Your teeth could become loose as the gums pull away from them.
- **Frequent gum disease/infection:** As well as the previous gum symptoms, you may experience more frequent gum disease and/or gum infections.
- **Sexual dysfunction among men:** If you are over 50 and experience frequent or constant sexual dysfunction *(erectile dysfunction)*, it could be a symptom of Diabetes.
- **Numbness or tingling, especially in your feet and hands:** If there is too much sugar in your body your nerves could become damaged, as could the tiny blood vessels that feed those nerves. You may experience tingling and/or numbness in your hands and feet.

Doctors can determine whether a patient has a normal metabolism, Pre-Diabetes or Diabetes in one of three different ways - there are three possible tests:

- The Fasting Plasma Glucose *(FPG)* test
- The A1C test
- The Oral Glucose Tolerance Test *(OGTT)*

The Fasting Plasma Glucose *(FPG)* test

Diabetes	
Fasting plasma glucose	≥ 7.0 mmol/L (126 mg/dl)
2-h plasma glucose *(Venous plasma glucose 2 hours after ingestion of 75 g oral glucose load)*	***or*** ≥ 11.1 mmol/L (200 mg/dl) ***or***
HbA1c	≥ 6.5%

Impaired glucose tolerance *(IGT)*	
Fasting plasma glucose	< 7.0 mmol/L (126 mg/dl)
2-h plasma glucose *(Venous plasma glucose 2 hours after ingestion of 75 g oral glucose load)*	***and*** ≥ 7.8 and < 11.1 mmol/L (140 mg/dl and 200 mg/dl)

Impaired fasting glucose *(IFG)*	
Fasting plasma glucose	6.1 to 6.9 mmol/L (110 mg/dl to 125 mg/dl)
2-h plasma glucose *(Venous plasma glucose 2 hours after ingestion of 75 g oral glucose load)*	***and*** *(if measured)* < 7.8 mmol/L (140 mg/dl)

Gestational Diabetes *(GDM)*	
One or more of the following:	
Fasting plasma glucose	5.1–6.9 mmol/L (92–125 mgl/dl)
1-h plasma glucose *(Venous plasma glucose 1 hour after ingestion of 75 g oral glucose load)*	≥ 10.0 mmol/L (180 mg/dl)
2-h plasma glucose	8.5–11.0 mmol/L (153–199 mg/dl)

The A1C test

A1C test is a measure of your average blood sugar over the previous 3 months. This test requires only a small amount of blood and no fasting.

➡ at least 6.5% means Diabetes

➡ between 5.7% and 5.99% means Pre-Diabetes

➡ less than 5.7% means normal

The Oral Glucose Tolerance Test *(OGTT)*

➡ at least 200 mg/dl means Diabetes

➡ between 140 and 199.9 mg/dl means Pre-Diabetes

➡ less than 140 mg/dl means normal

An abnormal reading following the OGTT means the patient has Impaired Glucose Tolerance *(IGT)*.

Although it is very important to mention that in people who do not have symptoms, a positive test for Diabetes should be repeated on another day.

Diabetes is a "*silent killer*". It feels and seems harmless, however any of the previously mentioned symptoms could lead to early death which you can avoid with a usually free blood sugar level test.

So if any of the main symptoms fits you it could be a life saving act to do the test for blood sugar level immediately, especially if you are experiencing Frequent urination, Disproportionate thirst, Intense hunger, Weight gain or Unusual weight loss.

Blood glucose measurement is relatively simple, cheap and should be available at primary health-care level. Not to mention that if you do not feel confident to visit a doctor, than you have many other options. For instance many stores selling Diabetes related products and various institutions offer free blood glucose testing.

For example the American wholesale chain CastCo offers free of charge Diabetes A1C tests in their healthcare clinics and pharmacies. This test requires only a small amount of blood and no fasting, and usually you have your result in seconds.

Facts & Myths *Nr 3.*

Myth: Fat people always develop Type 2 Diabetes eventually.

Fact: This is not true! Being overweight or obese raises the risk of becoming diabetic, they are risk factors, but do not mean that an obese person will definitely become diabetic.

Many people with Type 2 Diabetes were never overweight. The majority of overweight people do not develop Type 2 Diabetes.

Types of Diabetes

"IN THE GENERAL PUBLIC DIABETES OFTEN EQUALS WITH TYPE 2 DIABETES, ERGO IT IS ALL ABOUT BEING FAT. THIS IS A WRONG MISCONCEPTION."

Technically speaking the general public is aware of only three types of Diabetes *(Type 1, Type 2, Gestational Diabetes)*, however in reality we can define at least seven different types.

Especially since the word Diabetes refers both to Diabetes Insipidus and Diabetes Mellitus. They both have similar symptoms such as the increased thirst and frequent urination, however these are completely different in terms of mechanism.

Both cause large amounts of urine to be produced *(polyuria)*. However, Diabetes Insipidus is either a problem with the production of antidiuretic hormone *(Central Diabetes Insipidus)* or the kidney's response to antidiuretic hormone *(Nephrogenic Diabetes Insipidus)*, whereas Diabetes Mellitus causes polyuria via a process called osmotic diuresis, due to the high blood sugar leaking into the urine and taking excess water along with it.

Still, the main and most important distinction is that the urine of Diabetes Insipidus patients does not contain glucose.

For this reason we have to separate Diabetes Insipidus, which is caused by either hormonal or kidney problems from Diabetes Mellitus.

So let's see the six different types of Diabetes Mellitus:

- **Type 1**, is the juvenile Diabetes. It usually effects children in a very early age.
- **Type 1.5,** also called as LADA, is a form of Diabetes Type 1 that occurs in adults.
- **Pre-Diabetes**, when the blood glucose levels are high, but not high enough for a diagnosis of Type 2 Diabetes.
- **Type 2**, usually effects elderly and obese people.
- **Type 3**, is a proposed term for Alzheimer's disease resulting in an insulin resistance in the brain.
- **Gestational Diabetes**, which affects females during pregnancy.

Interestingly from the 422 million people all around the World suffering from Diabetes almost 90% has Type 2 Diabetes. And maybe this is the exact reason why many people have a wrong understanding about this complex disease.

In the general public Diabetes often equals with Type 2 Diabetes, ergo it is all about being fat. This is a wrong misconception.

It is even true for medical experts, since distinguishing between Type 1 Diabetes and Type 2 Diabetes is not always easy, as it often requires relatively sophisticated laboratory tests for pancreas function.

Facts & Myths *Nr 4.*

Myth: High blood sugar levels are fine for some, while for others they are a sign of Diabetes.

Fact: High blood-sugar levels are never normal for anybody. Some illnesses, mental stress and steroids can cause temporary hikes in blood sugar levels in people without Diabetes. Anybody with higher-than-normal blood sugar levels or sugar in their urine should be checked for Diabetes by a health care professional.

It is also the reason why distinct global estimates of Diabetes prevalence for Type 1 and Type 2 do not exist.

Type 1 Diabetes previously known as Insulin-Dependent Diabetes Mellitus *(IDDM)*, Juvenile or Childhood-onset Diabetes, is characterized by deficient insulin production in the body. Type 1 Diabetes results from the pancreas's failure to produce enough insulin. The cause is unknown.

People with Type 1 Diabetes always require daily administration of insulin to regulate the amount of glucose in their blood. If they do not have access to insulin, they cannot survive.

The cause of Type 1 Diabetes is not known and it is currently not preventable. Symptoms include excessive urination and thirst, constant hunger, weight loss, vision changes and fatigue.

Type 1.5 Diabetes, often called as **Latent Autoimmune Diabetes of Adults** *(LADA)*. It is a condition in which Type 1 Diabetes Mellitus develops in adults. Adults with LADA are frequently initially misdiagnosed as having Type 2 Diabetes Mellitus, based on age rather than etiology.

Pre-Diabetes indicates a condition that occurs when a person's blood glucose levels are higher than normal but not high enough for a diagnosis of Type 2 Diabetes Mellitus. Many people destined to develop Type 2 Diabetes Mellitus spend many years in a state of Pre-Diabetes.

It is very important to mention here two serious conditions, the **Impaired Glucose Tolerance** *(IGT)* and the **Impaired Fasting Glycaemia** *(IFG)*. They are both intermediate conditions in the transition between normal blood glucose levels and Diabetes *(especially Type 2)*, though the transition is not inevitable.

People with Impaired Glucose Tolerance or Impaired Fasting Glycaemia are at increased risk of heart attacks and strokes.

Type 2 Diabetes is formerly called Non-Insulin-Dependent or Adult-onset Diabetes, it results from the body's ineffective use of insulin.

Type 2 Diabetes accounts for the vast majority of people with Diabetes around the world.

The Type 2 Diabetes begins with insulin resistance in the body, a condition in which cells fail to respond to insulin properly. For this reason the symptoms may be similar to those of Type 1 Diabetes, but are often less marked or absent.

As a result, the disease may go undiagnosed for several years, until complications have already arisen.

While the cause of Type 1 Diabetes is still unknown, the primary cause of Type 2 Diabetes is excessive body weight and not enough exercise.

For many years **Type 2 Diabetes** was seen only in adults but it has **begun to occur in children**. Overweight and obesity are the strongest risk factors for Type 2 Diabetes.

Type 3 Diabetes is a proposed term for Alzheimer's disease resulting in an insulin resistance in the brain.

The discovery of the relation between the increased insulin resistance in the brain and the Alzheimer's is relatively new, only known since 2005.

Gestational Diabetes *(GDM)* is a temporary condition that occurs during pregnancy and carries long-term risk of Type 2 Diabetes.

The condition is present when blood glucose values are above normal but still below those diagnostic of Diabetes.

Women with gestational Diabetes are at increased risk of some complications during pregnancy and delivery, as are their infants.

Gestational Diabetes is diagnosed through prenatal screening, rather than reported symptoms.

Type 1 Diabetes

"IT IS ESTIMATED THAT ABOUT 80,000 CHILDREN DEVELOP THE DISEASE EACH YEAR.

12% OF PEOPLE WITH TYPE 1 DIABETES HAVE CLINICAL DEPRESSION."

When People are unable to produce insulin we are usually talking about Type 1 Diabetes *(T1D)*.

This can be a fatal state since the person's body has destroyed his/her own insulin-producing beta cells in the pancreas. Patients with Type 1 Diabetes regularly take exogenous insulin and will likely go into a coma if it is untreated.

Type 1 Diabetes is also known as Juvenile Diabetes or Childhood Diabetes. The reason for that is the fact that most of the Type 1 Diabetes patients develop the condition during childhood or teenage years. Although it can also develop after the age of 18 and before the age of 40, it is extremely rare to get Type 1 Diabetes by the age near 40.

Unlike the Type 2 Diabetes, the Type 1 Diabetes is not preventable. Approximately 10% of all people with Diabetes Mellitus have Type 1 Diabetes and the majority of people who develop Type 1 Diabetes are of normal weight and are otherwise healthy during onset. As a matter of fact unlike Type 2 Diabetes, the onset of Type 1 Diabetes is unrelated to lifestyle.

Comparison of Type 1 and Type 2 Diabetes		
	Type 1	***Type 2***
Onset	Sudden	Gradual
Age at onset	Mostly in children	Mostly in adults
Body size	Thin or normal	Often obese
Ketoacidosis	Common	Rare
Autoantibodies	Usually present	Absent
Endogenous insulin	Low or absent	Normal, decreased or increased
Concordance in identical twins	50 %	90 %
Prevalence	~10%	~90%

The sad thing is that the exact causes of Type 1 Diabetes are unknown. It is generally agreed that Type 1 Diabetes is the result of a complex interaction between genes and environmental factors, though no specific environmental risk factors have been shown to cause a significant number of cases.

Type 1 Diabetes can be partly inherited, with multiple genes, more than 50 genes are associated to Type 1 Diabetes, including certain HLA genotypes, known to influence the risk of Diabetes.

Despite the misbeliefs, Type 1 Diabetes can not be reversed by diet and exercise. This is quite understandable since the person has lost his/her insulin-producing beta cells, which can be considered as the complete failure of their organ, the pancreas.

Patients with Type 1 Diabetes will need to take insulin injections for the rest of their life. Also for this reason some people may refer to this type as Insulin-Dependent Diabetes.

Currently there are many ongoing researches and attempts to find ways of preventing or slowing down the progress of Type 1

Diabetes, but so far with no proven success. The only success which we can mention is that some patients have had their beta cells replaced through a pancreas transplant and have managed to produce their own insulin again.

It is interesting to mention that the World Health Organization *(WHO)* created a study which highlighted that Type 1 Diabetes is most common in Scandinavian populations and in Sardinia and Kuwait, and much less common in Asia and Latin America.

The first signs of having Type 1 Diabetes are the classical symptoms of polyuria *(frequent urination)*, polydipsia *(increased thirst)*, polyphagia *(increased hunger)*, xerostomia *(dry mouth)*, fatigue and weight loss.

About a quarter of people with new Type 1 Diabetics are diagnosed when they present with Diabetic Ketoacidosis. The signs and symptoms of Diabetic Ketoacidosis include xeroderma *(dry skin)*, rapid deep breathing, drowsiness, abdominal pain and vomiting.

Although the cause of Type 1 Diabetes Mellitus is unknown, it results from the autoimmune destruction of the insulin-producing beta cells in the pancreas.

Type 2 Diabetes is characterized by insulin resistance, while Type 1 Diabetes is characterized by insulin deficiency, generally without insulin resistance. The subsequent lack of insulin leads to increased glucose in blood and urine and administration of insulin is becoming essential for survival. Insulin therapy must be continued indefinitely and typically does not impair normal daily activities.

The devastating effect of Type 1 Diabetes on the body can be perfectly clearly presented with the shocking fact that about **12% of people with Type 1 Diabetes have clinical depression**.

Globally, the exact number of people with Type 1 Diabetes is unknown, it accounts approximately 10% of all Diabetes cases.

It is estimated that about 80,000 children develop the disease each year. The development of new cases vary by country and region; the lowest rates appear to be in Japan and China with approximately 1 person per 100,000 per year; the highest rates are found in Scandinavia where it is closer to 35 new cases per 100,000 per year. The United States and other countries in northern Europe fall somewhere in between with 8-17 new cases per 100,000 per year.

The cause of Type 1 Diabetes is unknown however number of explanatory theories have been put forward, and the cause may be one or more of the following:

➡ genetic susceptibility,

➡ a diabetogenic trigger, and/or

➡ exposure to an antigen.

Talking about **genetic susceptibility**, the risk of a child developing Type 1 Diabetes is about 10% if the father has it, about 10% if a sibling has it, about 4% if the mother has Type 1 Diabetes and was aged 25 or younger when the child was born, and about 1% if the mother was over 25 years old when the child was born.

Some research has suggested breastfeeding decreases the risk in later life.

> ***Facts & Myths*** *Nr 5.*
>
> *Myth:* Children can outgrow Diabetes.
>
> *Fact:* Unfortunately this is not true. Nearly all children with Diabetes have Type 1, therefore their insulin-producing beta cells in the pancreas have been destroyed. These never come back.
>
> Children with Type 1 Diabetes will need to take insulin for the rest of their lives, unless a cure is found one day.

Environmental factors can influence expression of Type 1 Diabetes. For identical twins, when one twin has Type 1 Diabetes, the other twin only has it 30%–50% of the time. Thus for 50%-70% of identical twins where one has the disease, the other will not, despite having exactly the same genome; this suggests environmental factors, in addition to genetic factors, can influence the disease's prevalence.

Other indications of environmental influence include the presence of a 10-fold difference in occurrence among Caucasians living in different areas of Europe, and that people tend to acquire the rate of disease of their particular destination country.

Also unforeseen circumstances or **increased stress can trigger the Type 1 Diabetes** in the patients. It is not unusual that the body is answering to extreme stress with a dramatic and lasting physical response such as Diabetes.

Trauma can affect our genes, even a simplest psychological stress may have a negative effect on Type 1 Diabetics.

Anxiety due to stress, causes many changes in the body because when there is physical or emotional stress the adrenal glands produce more of the hormones adrenaline and cortisol.

Adrenaline also raises blood sugar and tries to free up the energy we may need and in extreme circumstances our body can react with developing Diabetes.

Of course there are other theories as well taking away the responsibility from our environments.

One theory proposes that Type 1 Diabetes is a **virus-triggered autoimmune response** in which the immune system attacks virus-infected cells along with the beta cells in the pancreas. The **Coxsackie virus** family or **Rubella** is implicated, although the evidence is inconclusive.

This vulnerability is not shared by everyone, since not everyone infected by the suspected virus develops Type 1 Diabetes. This has suggested presence of a genetic vulnerability and there is indeed an observed inherited tendency to develop Type 1 Diabetes. It has been traced to particular HLA genotypes, though the connection between them and the triggering of an autoimmune reaction remains poorly understood.

Other theories suggest that pancreatic problems, including trauma, pancreatitis, or tumors *(either malignant or benign)* can also lead to loss of insulin production.

It is a more likely scenario especially since many drugs and chemicals can influence the reaction of the body. For example some chemicals and drugs selectively destroy pancreatic cells.

Just to ensure an example there is *(was)* Pyrinuron *(Vacor)*, a rodenticide introduced drug in the United States in 1976, that selectively destroys pancreatic beta cells, resulting in Type 1 Diabetes after ingestion. Pyrinuron was withdrawn from the U.S. market in 1979 but is still used in some countries.

Or there is Streptozotocin *(Zanosar)*, an antibiotic and antineoplastic agent used in chemotherapy for pancreatic cancer, which also kills beta cells resulting in loss of insulin production.

So let's face the facts that part of the Type 1 Diabetics are victims of the drugs and chemicals, however this is just the minority of the Type 1 patients.

We still do not know what triggers the disease in the children who probably never tasted these drugs and chemicals. And this is scary, leaving us with a disease which is not currently preventable.

So how is life with Type 1 Diabetes?

Diet with Type 1 Diabetes is relatively not bad.

Since Type 1 Diabetes is not related to your lifestyle, almost every food is welcomed until you measure and control the carbohydrates.

Luckily you do not need to restrict yourself to boring bland foods. Even sugary foods are acceptable if you include them in your food plan.

Generally speaking foods that are low in fat, salt and have no or very little added sugar are ideal. Just as for every healthy human being a diet that controls the person's blood sugar level as well as his/her blood pressure and cholesterol levels will help achieve the best possible health.

> ***Facts & Myths*** *Nr 6.*
>
> *Myth:* Do not eat too much sugar, you will become diabetic.
>
> *Fact:* This is not always true. A person with Type 1 Diabetes developed the disease because their immune system destroyed the insulin-producing beta cells.
>
> A diet high in calories, which can make people overweight/obese, raises the risk of developing Type 2 Diabetes, especially if there is a history of this disease in the family.

It is suggested to consume plenty of fruits, vegetables and whole grains - foods that are highly nutritious, low in fat, and low in calories. A low-carbohydrate diet, in addition to medications, is useful in Type 1 Diabetes.

The most important thing is that before every meal the Type 1 Diabetes patient needs to calculate the carbohydrates and adjust their insulin, so that the food and insulin can work together to control blood glucose levels.

Therefore the biggest change is that a person with Type 1 Diabetes always will have to watch what he/she eats.
Although it is not a mandatory thing a dietitian can help you create a food plan that suits you. Most dietitians agree that you should aim to consume the same quantity of food, with equal portions of carbs, proteins and fats at the same time each day.

Physical activity is highly recommended, Type 1 Diabetes patients must try to make physical activity part of their daily life routine. However there is a big difference between exercise and exercise. For this reason it is always good to consult with a doctor who can explain before starting exercising, whether that routine is really good or not.

For example climbing a mountain can increase your stress level which can influence your physical and mental balance. In general the physical activity or exercise for people with Type 1 Diabetes means aerobic exercise.

Many Type 1 Diabetes patients did not have any exercise before they were diagnosed, but still it is always good to build up gradually. Physical activity helps lower your blood sugar and make you fit and looks nice for your loved ones. Therefore its benefits are enormous for your physical and mental health.

Before any kind of physical activity it is highly important to understand that a person with Type 1 Diabetes has to manually adjust his/her insulin doses - the body will not respond automatically.

Remember to check your blood sugar level more frequently during your first few weeks of exercise so that you may adapt your meal plans and/or insulin doses accordingly.

Exercise will also help your circulation - helping to make sure your lower legs and feet are healthy, which is a very important thing for people with Diabetes.

Complications can be very serious with Type 1 Diabetes. A person with Type 1 Diabetes has four times higher risk of developing heart disease, stroke, high blood pressure, blindness, kidney failure, damage to the eyes, gum disease and nerve damage, compared to a person who does not have any type of Diabetes.

Talking about circulation in the body, a person with Type 1 Diabetes is more likely to have poor blood circulation through his/her legs and feet. If left untreated the problem may become such that a foot has to be amputated. Unfortunately it is a very likely issue with many people (*not*)fighting with Type 1 Diabetes.

People are usually trained to independently manage their Diabetes however for some this can be challenging, and untreated Diabetes can cause many complications.

Poorly managed Type 1 Diabetes can cause acute complications include Diabetic Ketoacidosis *(too high blood sugar level)* and Non-Ketotic Hyperosmolar Coma which can be fatal if untreated. Diabetic ketoacidosis can cause accumulation of liquid in the brain *(cerebral edema)*.

This is a life-threatening issue and children are at a higher risk for cerebral edema than adults, causing Ketoacidosis to be the most common cause of death in pediatric Diabetes.

The good news is that treatment is available and it is effective and can help prevent these complications from happening.

Here are **some tips for the preventions** of the problems:

- ✓ Keep your blood pressure under 130/85 mm Hg.
- ✓ Keep your cholesterol level below 200 mg.
- ✓ Check your feet every day for signs of infection.
- ✓ Get your eyes checked once a year.
- ✓ Get your dentist to check your teeth and gums twice a year.

And it might sound way too vulgar, but poorly treated Type 1 Diabetes can cause **sexual dysfunction**. In Diabetics sexual dysfunction is often a result of physical factors such as nerve damage and/or poor circulation, and psychological factors such as stress and/or depression caused by the demands of the disease. The most common sexual issues in Diabetic males are problems with erections and ejaculation.

While there is less material on the correlation between Diabetes and female sexual dysfunction than male sexual dysfunction, studies have shown there to be a significant prevalence of sexual problems in diabetic women. Common problems include reduced sensation in the genitals, dryness, difficulty/inability to orgasm, pain during sex, and decreased libido.

Women with Type 1 Diabetes show a higher than normal rate of polycystic ovarian syndrome *(PCOS)*.

Type 1.5 Diabetes (LADA)

> "IT IS ESTIMATED THAT MORE THAN 50% OF PERSONS DIAGNOSED AS HAVING NON-OBESITY-RELATED TYPE 2 DIABETES MAY ACTUALLY HAVE LADA."

LADA refers to Latent Autoimmune Diabetes of Adults. However you might also hear it as Late-onset Autoimmune Diabetes of Adulthood or Aging or Slow Onset Type 1 Diabetes.

Diabetes Type 1.5 is a form of Diabetes Mellitus Type 1 that occurs in adults, often with a slower course of onset. This is also the reason that often adults with LADA may initially be diagnosed as having Type 2 Diabetes based on their age. This particularly happens if they have risk factors for Type 2 Diabetes such as a strong family history or obesity.

The concept of Latent Autoimmune Diabetes Mellitus was first introduced in 1993 to describe Slow Onset Type 1 Autoimmune Diabetes in adults. This followed the concept that Glutamic Acid Decarboxylase Autoantibodies *(GADA)* were a feature of Type 1 Diabetes and not Type 2 Diabetes.

The symptoms of latent autoimmune Diabetes of adults are similar to those of other forms of Diabetes: such as excessive thirst and drinking, excessive urination, and often blurry vision.

Compared to childhood Type 1 Diabetes, the symptoms develop comparatively slowly.

It can only be treated with the usual oral treatments for Type 2 Diabetes for a certain period of time, after which insulin treatment is usually necessary, as well as long-term monitoring for complications.

Important facts on LADA

- **Onset:** Type 1 Diabetes onsets rapidly and at a younger age than does LADA.
- **Family history:** There is often a family history of autoimmune conditions. Contrary to popular belief, some people with latent autoimmune Diabetes of adults do carry a family history for Type 2 Diabetes.
- **Autoantibodies:** Persons with Type 1 Diabetes and LADA usually test positive for certain *(same)* autoantibodies *(GAD, ICA, IA-2, ZnT8)* that are not present in Type 2 Diabetes. Studies have reported an association of Type 1 Diabetes and LADA with high risk genes, HLA-DR3, HLA-DR4. There are also TCF7L2 genes associated with Type 2 Diabetes with latent autoimmune Diabetes of adults.
- **GAD autoantibodies:** Persons with LADA usually test positive for GAD antibodies, whereas in Type 1 Diabetes these antibodies are more commonly seen in adults rather than in children.
- **Insulin resistance:** People with LADA have insulin resistance similar to long-term Type 1 Diabetes; some studies showed that people with LADA have less insulin resistance, compared with those with Type 2 Diabetes; however, others have not found a difference.
- **Lifestyle and weight:** People with LADA typically have a normal BMI or may be underweight due to weight loss prior to diagnosis. Some people with LADA, however, may be overweight to mildly obese. LADA *(Type 1 Diabetes)* is an autoimmune disease that cannot be prevented.
- **Prognosis:** About 80% of all persons initially misdiagnosed with Type 2 Diabetes, who have GAD antibodies, will become insulin dependent within 3 to 15 years *(according to differing LADA sources)*. Those with both GAD and IA2 antibodies, however, will become insulin dependent sooner. LADA occurs more slowly than classic rapid-onset Type 1 Diabetes, though it progresses towards insulin dependency.

➡ **Treatment:** The treatment for Type 1 Diabetes and LADA is exogenous insulin, to control glucose levels, prevent further destruction of residual beta cells, reduce the possibility of diabetic complications, and prevent death from Diabetic Ketoacidosis *(DKA)*. Although LADA may appear to initially respond to similar treatment *(lifestyle and medications if needed)* as Type 2 Diabetes, it will not halt or slow the progression of beta cell destruction, and people with LADA will eventually become insulin dependent.

The diagnosis is based on the finding of high blood sugar together with the clinical impression that islet failure rather than insulin resistance is the main cause.

It is estimated that between 6-50% of all persons, depending on population, diagnosed with Type 2 Diabetes and shockingly more than **50% of persons diagnosed as having non-obesity-related Type 2 Diabetes may actually have LADA**.

Although it is incredible to say that the Expert Committee on the Diagnosis and Classification of Diabetes Mellitus does not recognize the term LADA; rather, it includes LADA in the definition of Type 1 autoimmune Diabetes.

It is important to note that not all people having LADA are thin or skinny, however there are overweight individuals with LADA who are misdiagnosed because of their weight.

Facts & Myths *Nr 7.*

Myth: People with Diabetes should not exercise.

Fact: Definitely not true! Exercise is important for people with Diabetes, as it is for everybody else.

Exercise helps manage body weight, improves cardiovascular health, improves mood, helps blood sugar control, and relieves stress. Patients should discuss exercise with their doctor first.

Moreover, it is now becoming evident that autoimmune Diabetes may be highly under-diagnosed in many individuals who have Diabetes, and that the body mass index levels may have rather limited use in connections with latent autoimmune Diabetes.

Glutamic acid decarboxylase autoantibody *(GADA)*, islet cell autoantibody *(ICA)*, insulinoma-associated *(IA-2)* autoantibody, and zinc transporter autoantibody *(ZnT8)* testing should be performed on all adults who are not obese who are diagnosed with Diabetes.

Detection of a low C-peptide and raised antibodies against the islets of Langerhans support the diagnosis.

Persons with LADA typically have low, although sometimes moderate, levels of C-peptide as the disease progresses.

Patients with insulin resistance or Type 2 Diabetes are more likely to, though will not always, have high levels of C-peptide due to an over production of insulin.

Glutamic Acid Decarboxylase Antibodies are commonly found in Type 1 Diabetes.

In addition to being useful in making an early diagnosis for Type 1 Diabetes, GADA tests are used for differential diagnosis between LADA and Type 2 Diabetes.

It may also be used for differential diagnosis of gestational Diabetes, risk prediction in immediate family members for Type 1 Diabetes, as well as a tool to monitor prognosis of the clinical progression of Type 1 Diabetes.

Pre-Diabetes

"PRE-DIABETES IS EFFECTING APPROXIMATELY 10%-15% OF ADULTS IN THE UNITED STATES."

Pre-Diabetes is the precursor stage to Diabetes Mellitus in which not all of the symptoms required to label a person as diabetic are present, but blood sugar is abnormally high. This stage is often referred to as the "*grey area*".

Metabolic syndrome and Pre-Diabetes may be the same disorder, just diagnosed by a different set of biomarkers.

When we are talking about Pre-Diabetes we usually refer to Impaired Fasting Glycaemia or Impaired Fasting Glucose *(IFG)* or Impaired Glucose Tolerance *(IGT)*.

Patients with Impaired Fasting Glucose have a condition in which the fasting blood glucose is elevated above what is considered normal levels but it is not high enough to be classified as Diabetes Mellitus.

While Impaired Glucose Tolerance is a Pre-Diabetic state of Hyperglycemia that is associated with insulin resistance.

These two conditions, the Impaired Fasting Glucose and Impaired Glucose Tolerance are effecting approximately 10%-15% of adults in the United States.

Impaired Fasting Glycaemia

The name IFG refers to Impaired Fasting Glycaemia or Impaired Fasting Glucose which is considered as a Pre-Diabetic state, because the fasting blood glucose is already and consistently elevated above the normal levels, but not high enough to be classified as Diabetes Mellitus.

This Pre-Diabetic state is associated with insulin resistance and increased risk of cardiovascular pathology, although of lesser risk than Impaired Glucose Tolerance *(IGT)*. However and still Impaired Fasting Glycaemia is also a risk factor for mortality.

> ***Facts & Myths*** *Nr 8.*
>
> *Myth:* "I know when my blood sugar levels are high or low."
>
> *Fact:* Very high or low blood sugar levels may cause some symptoms, such as weakness, fatigue and extreme thirst.
>
> However, levels need to be fluctuating a lot for symptoms to be felt. The only way to be sure about your blood sugar levels is to test them regularly.
>
> Researchers from the University of Copenhagen, Denmark showed that even very slight rises in blood-glucose levels significantly raise the risk of ischemic heart disease.

Among its signs and symptoms you can find sudden sweating, confusion, thirst, hunger, heart palpitations, impaired speech, difficulty focusing - these are just a few symptoms and are not just limited to these.

Having Impaired Fasting Glycaemia you have a 50% chance that it will progress into Type 2 Diabetes Mellitus within 2 to 10 years.

However the newest studies reveal that the average time for progression is less than three years.

As a Pre-Diabetic you might prevent Type 2 Diabetes if you are able to change on your lifestyle.

Fasting blood glucose levels are in a continuum within a given population, with higher fasting glucose levels corresponding to a higher risk for complications caused by the high glucose levels.

Some patients with Impaired Fasting Glucose may also be diagnosed with Impaired Glucose Tolerance, but many have normal responses to a glucose tolerance test.

Criteria defined by World Health Organization
fasting plasma glucose level from 6.1 mmol/l (110 mg/dL) *to* 6.9 mmol/L (125 mg/dL)

Criteria defined by American Diabetes Association
fasting plasma glucose level from 5.6 mmol/L (100 mg/dL) *to* 6.9 mmol/L (125 mg/dL)

It is interesting to observe that the World Health Organization *(WHO)* has a different criteria for impaired fasting glucose than the American Diabetes Association *(ADA)*. The reason of this lies in the definition of the normal range of glucose which is different by each.

The World Health Organization also opted to keep its upper limit of normal at under 6.1 mmol/l *(110 mg/dL)* for fear of causing too many people to be diagnosed as having impaired fasting glucose.

Impaired Glucose Tolerance

Impaired Glucose Tolerance *(IGT)* is a Pre-Diabetic state of Hyperglycemia that is associated with insulin resistance and increased risk of cardiovascular pathology.

According to the criteria of the World Health Organization and the American Diabetes Association, Impaired Glucose Tolerance is defined as:

> *Two-hour glucose levels of 140 to 199 mg per dL (7.8 to 11.0 mmol/l) on the 75-g oral glucose tolerance test. A patient is said to be under the condition of Impaired Glucose Tolerance when he/she has an intermediately raised glucose level after 2 hours, but less than the level that would qualify for Type 2 Diabetes Mellitus. The fasting glucose may be either normal or mildly elevated.*

Impaired Glucose Tolerance may precede Type 2 Diabetes Mellitus by many years. The risk of progression to Diabetes and development of cardiovascular disease is greater than for Impaired Fasting Glucose.

Impaired Glucose Tolerance is also a serious risk factor for mortality.

Although some drugs can delay the onset of Diabetes, lifestyle modifications play a greater role in the prevention of Diabetes.

Patients identified as having an Impaired Glucose Tolerance should exercise regularly, lose 5% to 7% of body weight, and limit Intake of *(at least)* sugar and highly processed carbohydrates.

Type 2 Diabetes

> "APPROXIMATELY 90% OF ALL CASES OF DIABETES WORLDWIDE ARE OF THIS TYPE."

Type 2 Diabetes is the most common type of Diabetes Mellitus, it is highly related to the lifestyle of the patient and approximately 90% of all cases of Diabetes worldwide are of this type.

Comparison of Type 1 and Type 2 Diabetes		
	Type 1	***Type 2***
Onset	Sudden	Gradual
Age at onset	Mostly in children	Mostly in adults
Body size	Thin or normal	Often obese
Ketoacidosis	Common	Rare
Autoantibodies	Usually present	Absent
Endogenous insulin	Low or absent	Normal, decreased or increased
Concordance in identical twins	50 %	90 %
Prevalence	~10%	~90%

The major difference between Type 1 Diabetes is that the pancreas is still working, so the organ never stopped producing insulin.

It can happen that the body does not produce enough insulin for proper function, or the cells in the body do not react to insulin *(insulin resistance)*, but still the organ, the pancreas is working.

Also it is an important difference that Type 2 Diabetes generally appears later on in life, compared to Type 1 Diabetes.

A person with Type 2 Diabetes either

- ➡ Does not produce enough insulin, or
- ➡ Suffers from 'insulin resistance', which means that the insulin is not working properly.

What is happening is that the defective responsiveness of body tissues to insulin is believed to involve the insulin receptor. However the specific defects are not known. Diabetes Mellitus cases due to a known defect are classified separately.

The World Health Organization definition of Diabetes *(both Type 1 Diabetes and Type 2 Diabetes)* is for a single raised glucose reading with symptoms, otherwise raised values on two occasions, of either:

Symptoms of Diabetes either

- ➡ fasting plasma glucose ≥ 7.0 mmol/l (126 mg/dl)

  or
- ➡ with a glucose tolerance test, two hours after the oral dose a plasma glucose ≥ 11.1 mmol/l (200 mg/dl)

Some people may be able to control their Type 2 Diabetes symptoms by losing weight, following a healthy diet, doing plenty of exercise, and monitoring their blood glucose levels.

However, **Type 2 Diabetes** is typically a **progressive disease** - it gradually gets worse - and the patient will probably end up have to take insulin, usually in tablet form.

Previously seen mainly in middle-aged and elderly people, Type 2 Diabetes **occurs increasingly** frequently **in children** and young people.

Type 2 Diabetes is often undiagnosed and studies to assess the number of newly occurring cases are complicated and consequently there are almost no data on true incidence. World Health Organization's recent review of data from seven countries found that between 24% and 62% of people with Diabetes were undiagnosed and untreated. This is a shockingly high number.

Overweight and obese people have a much higher risk of developing Type 2 Diabetes compared to those with a healthy body weight. People with a lot of visceral fat, also known as central obesity, belly fat, or abdominal obesity, are especially at risk.

Being overweight/obese causes the body to release chemicals that can destabilize the body's cardiovascular and metabolic systems.

But being overweighted might be a parental responsibility as well. **A simple blood test could predict whether children as young as five are at risk of becoming obese in later life.**

The test, which looks at a fat storage gene, will enable parents to change the lifestyles of children before the pounds pile on.

Although the risk of Type 2 Diabetes is determined by an interplay of genetic and metabolic factors, by being overweight, physically inactive and eating the wrong foods all contribute to our risk of developing Type 2 Diabetes. Ethnicity, family history of Diabetes, and previous gestational Diabetes combined with older age, overweight and obesity, unhealthy diet, physical inactivity and smoking increase risk.

Drinking just one can of *(non-diet)* soda per day can raise our risk of developing Type 2 Diabetes by 22%, researchers from Imperial College London reported in the journal Diabetologia.

Scientists believe that the impact of sugary soft drinks on Diabetes risk may be a direct one, rather than simply an influence on body weight.

The fundings were so serious that in January 2014 Mexico implemented a nationwide tax on drinks containing added sugar.

The risk of developing Type 2 Diabetes is also greater as we get older. Experts are not completely sure why, but they say that as we age we tend to put on weight and become less physically active.

Those with a close relative who have/had Type 2 Diabetes, people of Middle Eastern, African, or South Asian descent also have a higher risk of developing the disease.

Also the older you are the higher your risk is, especially if you are over 40 *(for white people)*, and over 25 *(for black, South Asian and some minority groups)*. It has been found in the UK that black people and people of South Asian origin have five times the risk of developing Type 2 Diabetes compared to white people.

Excess body fat, overweight and obesity, together with physical inactivity, are estimated to cause a large proportion of the global Diabetes burden. Higher waist circumference and higher Body Mass Index *(BMI)* are associated with increased risk of Type 2 Diabetes.

Of course this may vary in different populations for example populations in South-East Asia develop Diabetes at a lower level of Body Mass Index than populations of European origin.

Several dietary practices are linked to unhealthy body weight and/or Type 2 Diabetes risk, including high intake of saturated fatty acids, high total fat intake and inadequate consumption of dietary beverages.

High intake of sugar-sweetened beverages, which contain considerable amounts of free sugars, increases the likelihood of being overweight or obese, particularly among children.

> ***Facts & Myths** Nr 9.*
>
> *Myth:* Only older people develop Type 2 Diabetes.
>
> *Fact:* Things are changing. A growing number of children and teenagers are developing Type 2 Diabetes. Experts say that this is linked to the explosion in childhood obesity rates, poor diet, and physical inactivity.

Early childhood nutrition affects the risk of Type 2 Diabetes later in life. Factors that appear to increase risk include poor fetal growth, low birth weight *(particularly if followed by rapid postnatal catch-up growth)* and high birth weight.

Active *(as distinct from passive)* smoking increases the risk of Type 2 Diabetes, with the highest risk among heavy smokers. Risk remains elevated for about 10 years after smoking cessation, falling more quickly for lighter smokers.

Men whose testosterone levels are low have been found to have a higher risk of developing Type 2 Diabetes. Researchers from the University of Edinburgh, Scotland, say that low testosterone levels are linked to insulin resistance.

However when you are getting older and you experience that your eyesight and hearing might not be as sharp as they were in your youth, Type 2 Diabetes can be the underlying reason.

It is always worth to check yourself for Diabetes Mellitus if you experience any of these five symptoms:

- ➡ You find it tougher to see or hear clearly
- ➡ You feel tired and grouchy
- ➡ You are experiencing odd symptoms
- ➡ You feel hungry all the time
- ➡ You urinate frequently and always feel thirsty

These symptoms are not necessarily present only because of your age. For example hearing loss is twice as common in people with diabetes as in those who do not have the disease.

Even if you are always tired can mean that your body is not effectively converting glucose to energy. Or a dry skin or tingling and numbness of the hands and feet can be the first warning sign.

Luckily **Type 2 Diabetes is preventable**. Regular physical activity reduces the risk of Type 2 Diabetes and raised blood glucose, and is an important contributor to overall energy balance, weight control and obesity prevention – all risk exposures linked to future Diabetes prevalence.

In the early stage of Type 2 Diabetes, the predominant abnormality is reduced insulin sensitivity. At this stage, high blood sugar can be reversed by a variety of measures and medications that improve insulin sensitivity or reduce the liver's glucose production.

However, the prevalence of physical inactivity globally is of increasing concern.

In 2010, *(the latest year for which data are available)* just under a quarter of all adults aged over 18 years did not meet the minimum recommendation for physical activity per week and were classified as insufficiently physically active.

Being overweight or obese is strongly linked to Type 2 Diabetes. Physical inactivity is alarmingly common among adolescents, with 84% of girls and 78% of boys not meeting minimum requirements for physical activity for this age.

Also women were more overweight or obese than men.
The prevalence of obesity was highest in the World Health Organization region of the Americas and lowest in the World Health Organization South-East Asian region.

Excess body fat is associated with 30% of cases in those of Chinese and Japanese descent, 60–80% of cases in those of European and African descent, and 100% of Pima Indians and Pacific Islanders.

Overall, despite the global voluntary target to halt the rise in obesity by 2025, being overweight or obese has increased in almost all countries.

The proportion of people who are overweight or obese increases with country income level.

High- and middle-income countries have more than double the overweight and obesity prevalence of low-income countries.

Management of Type 2 Diabetes focuses on lifestyle interventions, lowering other cardiovascular risk factors, and maintaining blood glucose levels in the normal range.

As for **medications** the patient will usually be prescribed orally administered anti-diabetic drugs. As a person with Type 2 Diabetes does produce his/her own insulin, a combination of oral medicines will usually improve insulin production, regulate the release of glucose by the liver, and treat insulin resistance to some extent.

If the beta cells become further impaired the patient will eventually need insulin therapy in order to regulate glucose levels.

No major Diabetes organization recommends universal screening for Diabetes as there is no evidence that such a program improve outcomes.

Also screening can be recommended among those whose blood pressure is less, who are overweight and between the ages of 40 and 70.

Type 3 Diabetes (Alzheimer's)

"DIABETES MEDICATION COULD TREAT ALZHEIMER'S!"

Type 3 Diabetes is a title that has been proposed for Alzheimer's disease which results from resistance to insulin in the brain. Type 3 Diabetes which is regarded as "*brain*" specific Diabetes is a dangerous Diabetes hybrid that was first discovered in 2005.

Studies carried out by the research team at Warren Alpert Medical School at Brown University identified the possibility of a new form of Diabetes after finding that insulin resistance can occur in the brain. The researchers pinpoint resistance to insulin and insulin-like growth factor as being a key part of the progression of Alzheimer's disease.

When it comes to the body, insulin is responsible for helping to convert food to energy. **The brain uses insulin too**, and it is believed that insulin's primary purpose in the brain is **to form memories** at synapses *(the spaces where cells in the brain communicate)*. Neurons save space for insulin receptors; insulin makes way for memories to form. In order for the brain to keep making more brain cells, it needs insulin.

A problem with insulin production in the brain is thought to result in the formation of protein "*plaque*", not unlike that which is found among sufferers of Type 1 Diabetes *(insulin-dependant)* and Type 2 Diabetes *(insulin-resistant)*. But in the case of Type 3 Diabetes, plaque appears in the brain and leads to memory loss and problems forming memories.

In short, the brain does not receive the energy it needs to form memories.

Researchers have discovered that many Type 2 Diabetics have deposits of a protein called amyloid beta in their pancreas, which is similar to the protein deposits found in the brain tissue of Alzheimer's sufferers.

As a conclusion people over the age of 60 who have insulin resistance, in particular those with Type 2 Diabetes have an increased risk of suffering from Alzheimer's disease, estimated to be between 50% and 65% higher.

In fact, it has been proposed that Alzheimer's disease could be known as Type 3 Diabetes, because insulin resistance in the brain is a key part of its progression.

Diabetes is also linked to memory loss more generally. Over time, the prolonged exposure to high blood glucose levels - caused by a lack of insulin production or ineffective insulin - can damage the hippocampus, which is the part of the brain that deals with concentration, attention, memory, and information processing.

Nobody knows exactly why Type 2 Diabetes increases the risk of Alzheimer's disease. Some research indicates that it is due to damage to the small blood vessels that feed cells and nerves caused by Diabetes.

According to a research team at Northwestern University, insulin may prevent or slow memory loss among those with Alzheimer's disease by protecting the synapses that form memory. Those with the disease tend to have lower insulin levels and are insulin-resistant.

The team found that the reason memory fails when insulin shortage occurs is because Amyloid beta-Derived Diffusible Ligands *(ADDLs)* destroy the receptors in the brain that typically are reserved for insulin, thus making the receptors insulin-resistant. Without the space for insulin, receptors cannot connect, and memory loss occurs.

In the past years researchers also discovered that **Diabetes medication could treat Alzheimer's**.

Researchers are also testing Diabetes medication as potential treatments for the neurodegenerative disease.

As it is today, Diabetes Type 3 is not completely understood. Diagnosis and treatments remain in the early stages, and mores studies are required in order to fully understand how to help those with Diabetes Type 3 Diabetes, as well as its connection to Alzheimer's and dementia.

Gestational Diabetes

"RISK FACTOR: UP TO ONE IN FOUR PREGNANCIES! DEPENDING ON THE REGION."

Gestational Diabetes Mellitus *(GDM)* is the one which affects females during pregnancy. It is typically diagnosed during the pregnancy and the majority of women can control it simply with exercise and diet.

Gestational Diabetes generally has few symptoms and it is most commonly diagnosed by screening during pregnancy. Diagnostic tests detect inappropriately high levels of glucose in blood samples.

Gestational Diabetes resembles Type 2 Diabetes in several respects, however **typically it will disappear after the baby is born**.

In most of cases *(75–90%)*, Gestational Diabetes is a condition in which women without previously diagnosed Diabetes exhibit high blood glucose *(blood sugar)* levels during pregnancy *(especially during their third trimester)*.

Gestational Diabetes is caused by improper insulin responses. This is likely due to pregnancy-related factors such as the presence of human placental lactogen that interferes with susceptible insulin receptors. This in turn causes inappropriately elevated blood sugar levels.

Scientists from the National Institutes of Health and Harvard University published a very interesting study whereby they found that women whose diets before becoming pregnant were high in animal fat and cholesterol had a higher risk for gestational Diabetes, compared to their counterparts whose diets were low in cholesterol and animal fats.

Typical risk factors and risk markers for women:

- age *(the older a woman of reproductive age is, the higher her risk of Gestational Diabetes)*
- overweight or obesity
- excessive weight gain during pregnancy
- a family history of Diabetes
- Gestational Diabetes during a previous pregnancy
- a history of stillbirth or giving birth to an infant with congenital abnormality
- and excess glucose in urine during pregnancy

The frequency of previously undiagnosed Diabetes in pregnancy and gestational Diabetes varies among populations but probably **affects** 10–25% of pregnancies, which means **up to one in four pregnancy**.

It has been estimated that most *(75–90%)* cases of high blood glucose during pregnancy are gestational Diabetes.

Some women have very high levels of glucose in their blood, and their bodies are unable to produce enough insulin to transport all of the glucose into their cells, resulting in progressively rising levels of glucose.

Between 10% to 20% of pregnant women with Gestational Diabetes will need to take some kind of blood-glucose-controlling medications.

Undiagnosed or uncontrolled Gestational Diabetes can raise the risk of complications during childbirth. As with Diabetes Mellitus in pregnancy in general, babies born to mothers with untreated gestational Diabetes are typically at increased risk of problems such as being large for gestational age *(which may lead to delivery complications)*, low blood sugar, and jaundice.

If untreated, it can also cause seizures or stillbirth. Not to mention the direct risk for the infant, since the baby can be bigger than he/she should be.

Generally speaking the Diabetes in pregnancy and Gestational Diabetes increase the risk of future obesity and Type 2 Diabetes in offspring.

However Gestational Diabetes is a treatable condition and in 90% of the cases women can control it simply with exercise and diet. The food plan is often the first recommended target for strategic management of Gestational Diabetes.

Treatment of Gestational Diabetes is also important because women with unmanaged Gestational Diabetes are at increased risk of developing Type 2 Diabetes Mellitus *(or very rarely, LADA or Type 1)* after pregnancy.

A woman is diagnosed with Gestational Diabetes when glucose intolerance continues beyond 24–28 weeks of gestation.

There is also a classification available for Gestational Diabetes, called "White classification". It was named after Priscilla White who pioneered research on the effect of Diabetes types on perinatal outcome, it is widely used to assess maternal and fetal risk.

The White classification distinguishes between Gestational Diabetes *(Type A)* and Pre-Gestational Diabetes *(Diabetes that existed prior to pregnancy)*.

These two groups are further subdivided according to their associated risks and management.

The **two subtypes of Gestational Diabetes** under this classification system are:

- **Type A1**: abnormal Oral Glucose Tolerance Test *(OGTT)*, but normal blood glucose levels during fasting and two hours after meals; diet modification is sufficient to control glucose levels.
- **Type A2**: abnormal Oral Glucose Tolerance Test compounded by abnormal glucose levels during fasting and/

or after meals; additional therapy with insulin or other medications is required.

Diabetes which **existed prior to pregnancy** is also split up into several subtypes under this system:

- **Type B**: onset at age 20 or older and duration of less than 10 years.
- **Type C**: onset at age 10–19 or duration of 10–19 years.
- **Type D**: onset before age 10 or duration greater than 20 years.
- **Type E**: overt Diabetes Mellitus with calcified pelvic vessels.
- **Type F**: diabetic nephropathy.
- **Type R**: proliferative retinopathy.
- **Type RF**: retinopathy and nephropathy.
- **Type H**: ischemic heart disease.
- **Type T**: prior kidney transplant.

An early age of onset or long-standing disease comes with greater risks, hence the first three subtypes.

The precise mechanisms underlying Gestational Diabetes remain unknown. The hallmark of Gestational Diabetes is increased insulin resistance. Pregnancy hormones and other factors are thought to interfere with the action of insulin as it binds to the insulin receptor. The interference probably occurs at the level of the cell signaling pathway behind the insulin receptor.

Since insulin promotes the entry of glucose into most cells, insulin resistance prevents glucose from entering the cells properly. As a result, glucose remains in the bloodstream, where glucose levels rise. More insulin is needed to overcome this resistance; about 1.5–2.5 times more insulin is produced than in a normal pregnancy.

Though the clinical presentation of Gestational Diabetes is well characterized, the biochemical mechanism behind the disease is not well known.

It is unclear why some women are unable to balance insulin needs and develop Gestational Diabetes; however a number of explanations have been given, similar to those in Type 2 Diabetes: autoimmunity, single gene mutations, obesity, along with other mechanisms.

A number of screening and diagnostic tests have been used to look for high levels of glucose in plasma or serum in defined circumstances.

One method is a stepwise approach where a suspicious result on a screening test is followed by diagnostic test.

Alternatively, a more involved diagnostic test can be used directly at the first prenatal visit for a woman with a high-risk pregnancy.

Non-challenge blood glucose tests involve measuring glucose levels in blood samples without challenging the subject with glucose solutions.

A blood glucose level is determined when fasting, 2 hours after a meal, or simply at any random time. In contrast, challenge tests involve drinking a glucose solution and measuring glucose concentration thereafter in the blood; in Diabetes, they tend to remain high.

The glucose solution has a very sweet taste which some women find unpleasant; sometimes, therefore, artificial flavours are added. Some women may experience nausea during the test, and more so with higher glucose levels.

Criteria for diagnosis of Gestational Diabetes, using the 100 gram Glucose Tolerance Test, according to Carpenter and Coustan:

Gestational Diabetes *(Carpenter and Coustan)*

- ➡ Fasting blood glucose level ≥95 mg/dl (5.33 mmol/L)
- ➡ 1 hour blood glucose level ≥180 mg/dl (10 mmol/L)
- ➡ 2 hour blood glucose level ≥155 mg/dl (8.6 mmol/L)
- ➡ 3 hour blood glucose level ≥140 mg/dl (7.8 mmol/L)

Criteria for diagnosis of gestational Diabetes according to National Diabetes Data Group:

Gestational Diabetes *(National Diabetes Data Group)*

- ➡ Fasting blood glucose level ≥105 mg/dl (5.8 mmol/L)
- ➡ 1 hour blood glucose level ≥190 mg/dl (10.6 mmol/L)
- ➡ 2 hour blood glucose level ≥165 mg/dl (9.2 mmol/L)
- ➡ 3 hour blood glucose level ≥145 mg/dl (8.1 mmol/L)

The glucose values used to detect Gestational Diabetes were first determined by O'Sullivan and Mahan *(1964)* in a retrospective cohort study *(using a 100 grams of glucose OGTT)* designed to detect risk of developing Type 2 Diabetes in the future.

The values were set using whole blood and required two values reaching or exceeding the value to be positive. Subsequent information led to alterations in O'Sullivan's criteria. When methods for blood glucose determination changed from the use of whole blood to venous plasma samples, the criteria for Gestational Diabetes were also changed.

And finally a very important thing to remember. It is a proven fact that Gestational Diabetes **signals future Diabetes** risk not only in mothers, but **also in fathers**.

The role of our Pancreas

"INSULIN IS PRODUCED IN THE PANCREAS. WITHOUT INSULIN THE GLUCOSE CANNOT ENTER OUR CELLS."

The pancreas is an important organ, part of our digestive system. Insulin is produced in the pancreas, when protein is ingested insulin is released.

The pancreas has two principal functions:

- ➡ It produces pancreatic digestive juices.
- ➡ It produces insulin and other digestive hormones.

The endocrine pancreas is the part of the pancreas that produces insulin and other hormones and the exocrine pancreas is the part of the pancreas that produces digestive juices.

Insulin is also released when glucose is present in the blood, without glucose in our cells they would not be able to function. After eating carbohydrates, blood glucose levels rise and insulin makes it possible for glucose to enter our body's cells. Without insulin the glucose cannot enter our cells.

The word pancreas comes from the Greek pankreas, meaning sweetbread.

It is located high up in your abdomen and lies across your body where the ribs meet at the bottom. It is shaped like a leaf and is about six inches *(16.5 cm)* long. The wide end is called the head while the narrower end is called the tail, the mid-part is called the body.

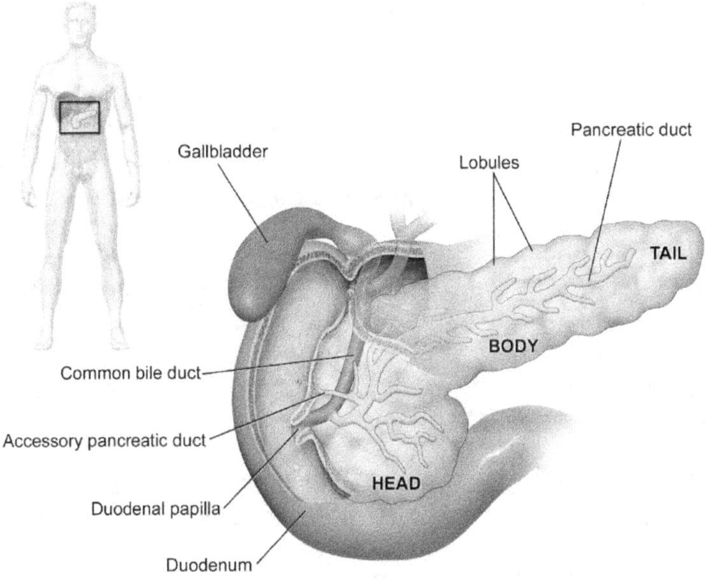

Photo credit: Blausen.com/WikiPedia

It is said that the pancreas was described first by Herophilus of Chalcedon in about 300 B.C. and the organ was named by Rufus of Ephesus in about 100 A.D. However, it is an established fact that the word pancreas had been used by Aristotle *(384-322B.C.)* before Herophilus.

In Aristotle's Historia Animalium, there is a line saying "*another to the so-called pancreas*". It is considered that the words "*so-called pancreas*" imply that the word pancreas had been popular at the time of Aristotle, but it had not been authorized yet as an anatomical term. However, the word pancreas presumably has been accepted as an anatomical term since Herophilus.

The Islets of Langerhans was discovered in 1869 by an anatomist named Paul Langerhans. He identified the keys cells in the pancreas which produce the main substance that controls glucose levels in the body.

The Islets of Langerhans contain Beta cells, which synthesize *(make)* the insulin. Approximately 1 to 3 million Islets of Langerhans make up the endocrine part of the pancreas *(mainly the exocrine gland)*, representing just one fiftieth of the pancreas' total mass.

The discovery of a role for the pancreas in Diabetes is generally ascribed to Joseph von Mering and Oskar Minkowski, who in 1889 found that dogs whose pancreas was removed developed all the signs and symptoms of Diabetes and died shortly afterwards.

In 1910, Sir Edward Albert Sharpey-Schafer suggested that people with Diabetes were deficient in a single chemical that was normally produced by the pancreas, he proposed calling this substance insulin, from the Latin insula, meaning island, in reference to the insulin-producing islets of Langerhans in the pancreas.

The endocrine role of the pancreas in metabolism, and indeed the existence of insulin, was further clarified in 1921, when Sir Frederick Grant Banting and Charles Herbert Best repeated the work of Von Mering and Minkowski, and went further to demonstrate they could reverse induced Diabetes in dogs by giving them an extract from the pancreatic islets of Langerhans of healthy dogs.

An effective treatment was only developed after the Canadians Frederick Banting and Charles Best first used insulin in 1921 and 1922.

What is Insulin?

> "INJECTIONS OF INSULIN ARE NECESSARY FOR THOSE LIVING WITH TYPE 1 DIABETES BECAUSE IT CANNOT BE TREATED BY DIET AND EXERCISE ALONE."

Insulin is a principal hormone produced by our pancreas which makes our body's cells absorb glucose from the blood. It regulates of the uptake of glucose from the blood into most cells of the body, especially liver, muscle, and adipose tissue and stops the body from using fat as a source of energy. Therefore deficiency of insulin or the insensitivity of its receptors plays a central role in all forms of Diabetes Mellitus.

The body obtains glucose from three main places:

- the intestinal absorption of food,
- the breakdown of glycogen, the storage form of glucose found in the liver,
- and gluconeogenesis, the generation of glucose from non-carbohydrate substrates in the body.

Insulin plays a critical role in balancing glucose levels in the body. Insulin can inhibit the breakdown of glycogen or the process of gluconeogenesis, it can stimulate the transport of glucose into fat and muscle cells, and it can stimulate the storage of glucose in the form of glycogen. Also **without insulin the body uses fat as a source of energy**.

Insulin is released into the blood by beta cells *(β-cells)*, found in the islets of Langerhans in the pancreas, in response to rising levels of blood glucose, typically after eating. Insulin is used by about two-thirds of the body's cells to absorb glucose from the blood for use as fuel, for conversion to other needed molecules, or for storage. Lower glucose levels result in decreased insulin release from the beta cells and in the breakdown of glycogen to glucose. This process is mainly controlled by the hormone glucagon, which acts in the opposite manner to insulin.

Effect of insulin on glucose uptake and metabolism

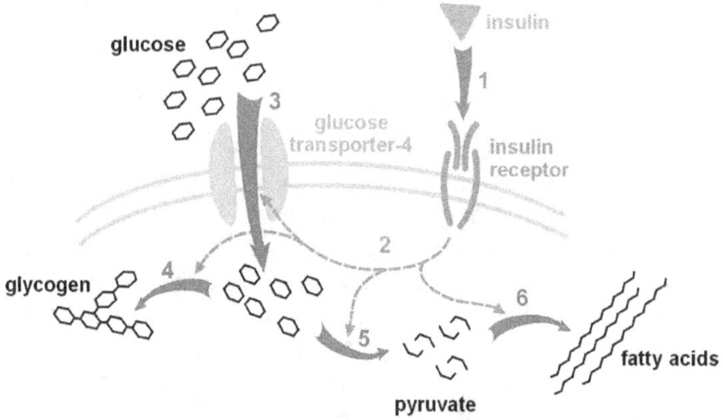

Photo credit: WikiPedia

If the amount of insulin available is insufficient, if cells respond poorly to the effects of insulin *(insulin insensitivity or insulin resistance)*, or if the insulin itself is defective, then glucose will not be absorbed properly by the body cells that require it, and it will not be stored appropriately in the liver and muscles. The net effect is persistently high levels of blood glucose, poor protein synthesis, and other metabolic derangements, such as acidosis.

When the glucose concentration in the blood remains high over time, the kidneys will reach a threshold of reabsorption, and glucose will be excreted in the urine *(glycosuria)*. This increases the osmotic pressure of the urine and inhibits reabsorption of water by the kidney, resulting in increased urine production *(polyuria)* and increased fluid loss. Lost blood volume will be replaced osmotically from water held in body cells and other body compartments, causing dehydration and increased thirst *(polydipsia)*.

There are four main **types of insulin**:

➡ **rapid acting** insulin: is used as a bolus dosage. The action onsets in 15 minutes with peak actions in 30 to 90 minutes.

➡ **short acting** insulin: action onsets within 30 minutes with the peak action around 2 to 4 hours.

➡ **intermediate** acting insulin: action onsets within 1 to 2 hours with peak action of 4 to 10 hours.

➡ **long acting** insulin: is usually given once per day.

In addition to insulin therapy dietary management is important. Injections of insulin either via subcutaneous injection or insulin pump are necessary for those living with Type 1 Diabetes because it cannot be treated by diet and exercise alone.

Although insulin is not identical in all the animal, **humans can receive animal insulin**. The porcine insulin, which is insulin from a pig is the most similar to human insulin and genetic engineering has allowed us to synthetically produce "*human*" insulin.

Today, the most common insulins are biosynthetic products produced using genetic recombination techniques; formerly, cattle or pig insulins were used, and even sometimes insulin from fish.

Discovery of insulin

The discovery of insulin is related to Dr. Frederick Banting *(November 14, 1891 – February 21, 1941)* who was a Canadian medical scientist, physician, painter and Nobel laureate noted as the first person to use insulin on humans.

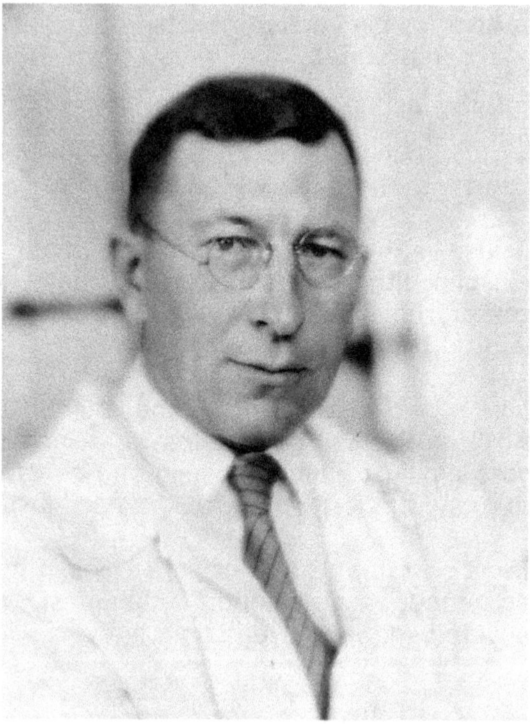

Photo credit: Library and Archives of Canada/WikiPedia

An article he read about the pancreas piqued Banting's interest in Diabetes. Banting had to give a talk on the pancreas to one of his classes at Western University on November 1, 1920, and he was therefore reading reports that other scientists had written. Although attempts to extract insulin from ground-up pancreas cells were unsuccessful, likely because of the destruction of the insulin by the proteolysis enzyme of the pancreas. The challenge was to find a way to extract insulin from the pancreas prior to it being destroyed.

Moses Barron published an article in 1920 which described experimental closure of the pancreatic duct by ligature, this further influenced Banting's thinking. The procedure caused deterioration of the cells of the pancreas that secrete trypsin, but left the islets of Langerhans intact.

Banting realized that this procedure would destroy the trypsin-secreting cells but not the insulin. Once the trypsin-secreting cells had died, insulin could be extracted from the islets of Langerhans.

Banting discussed this approach with J. J. R. Macleod, Professor of Physiology at the University of Toronto. Macleod provided experimental facilities and the assistance of one of his students, Dr. Charles Best. Banting and Best, with the assistance of biochemist James Collip, began the production of insulin by this means in 1921.

Their method involved tying a string around the pancrease duct. When examined several weeks later, the pancreatic digestive cells had died and been absorbed by the immune system. The process left behind thousands of islets. They isolated the extracts from the islets and produced isletin. What they called isletin became known as insulin.

Banting and Best managed to test this extract on dogs that had Diabetes. They discovered insulin. In fact, they managed to keep a dog, that had had its pancreas taken out alive throughout the whole summer by administering it the extract *(which was, in fact, insulin)*. The extract regulated the dogs blood sugar levels.

At this point, Professor J. MacLeod, who had placed the laboratory at their disposal, said he wanted to see a re-run of the whole trial. After doing so he decided to get his whole research team to work on the production and purification of insulin.

J.B. Collip joined the scientific team, which consisted of Banting, Best, Collip and MecLeod. They managed to produce enough insulin, in a pure enough form to be able to test it on patients.

In 1922 the insulin was tested on Leonard Thompson, a 14-year-old Diabetes patient who lay dying at the Toronto General Hospital. When he was given the insulin extract on January 23, his ketonuria and glycosuria were almost eliminated. His blood sugar levels dropped as low as 77%. At first he suffered a severe allergic reaction and further injections were cancelled.

The scientists worked hard on improving the extract and then a second dose of injections were administered on Thompson. The results were spectacular.

Six more patients were treated in February 1922 and quickly experienced an improved standard of life.

The scientists went to the other wards with diabetic children, most of them comatose and dying from Diabetic Ketoacidosis.

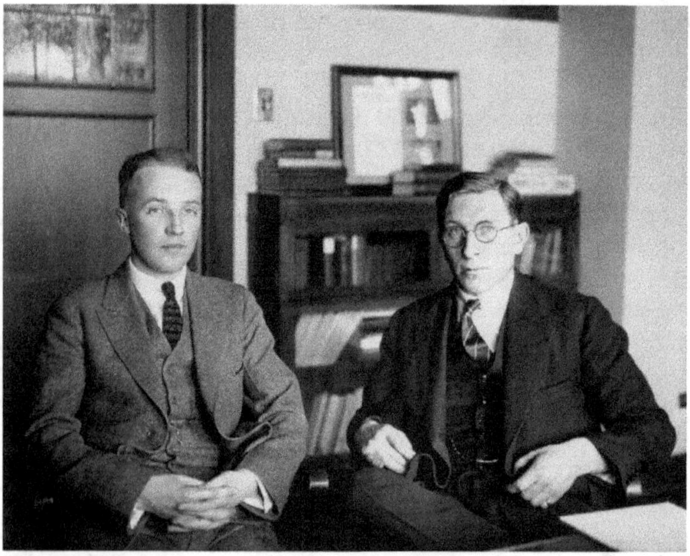

Dr. Frederick Banting with Charles H. Best
Photo credit: Library and Archives of Canada/WikiPedia

They went from bed-to-bed and injected them with the new purified extract - insulin. This is known as one of medicines most dramatic moments. Before injecting the last comatose children, the first started to awaken from their comas. A joyous moment for family members and hospital staff!

Collip did not get on too well with Banting and Best apparently and he soon left the project. Best continued trying to improve the extract and managed eventually to produce enough for the hospital's demand. Their work was privately published.

The Eli Lilly Company soon got to hear about it and offered to assist. It was not long before the Eli Lilly Company managed to produce large quantities of refined pure insulin.

In 1923 Banting and Macleod were awarded the Nobel Prize in Physiology or Medicine. Banting shared his prize with Best and Macleod shared his with Collip. **The patent for insulin was sold to the University of Toronto for one dollar.**

Banting and Best made the patent available without charge and did not attempt to control commercial production. Insulin production and therapy rapidly spread around the world, largely as a result of this decision.

Banting is honored by World Diabetes Day which is held on his birthday, November 14.

In 1994 Banting was inducted into the Canadian Medical Hall of Fame.

Also **a time capsule was placed in the Sir Frederick Banting Square in 1991 to honour the 100th anniversary of Sir Frederick Banting's birth. It was buried by the International Diabetes Federation Youth Representatives and Governor General Ray Hnatyshyn. It will be dug up when a cure for Diabetes is found.**

Inhalable insulin

Inhalable insulin is a powdered form of insulin, delivered with a nebulizer into the lungs where it is absorbed.

Insulin was introduced by Banting and Best from the University of Toronto in 1921 as an injectable agent however German researchers first introduced the idea of inhalable insulin already in 1924.

Years of failure followed until scientists realized they might be able to use new technologies to turn insulin into a concentrated powder with particles sized for inhalation.

In the 1980s Nektar Therapeutics developed technology to make insulin into small particles that they licensed to Pfizer. Alkermes developed a delivery device that they licensed to Eli Lilly and Company. Once concrete methods were developed, human tests began in the late 1990s.

In January 2006, the U.S. Food and Drug Administration *(FDA)* approved the use of Exubera, a form of inhalable insulin developed by Pfizer. It was approved in the UK in August 2006 but reimbursed by the National Health Service only for people who had problems with needles.

A 2007 systematic review concluded that the inhaled hexameric insulin Exubera *"appears to be as effective, but no better than injected short-acting insulin. The additional cost is so much more that it is unlikely to be cost-effective."*

However, in 2007, Pfizer announced that it would no longer manufacture or market Exubera. According to Chairman and CEO Jeffrey Kindler this was because Exubera *"failed to gain acceptance among patients and physicians."*

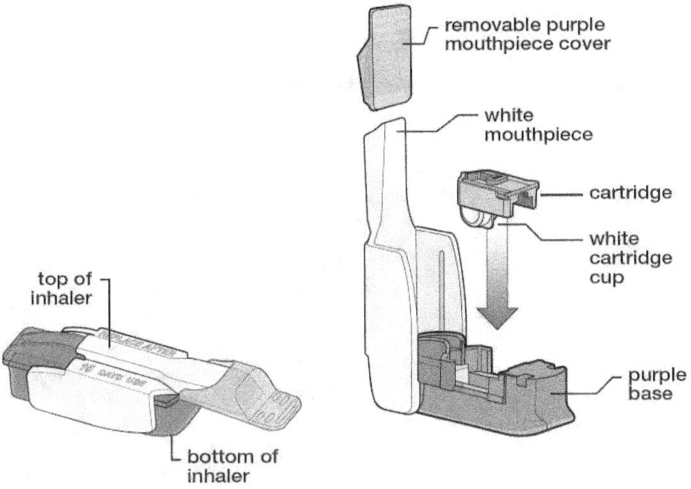

Photo credit: Afrezza/Mannkind

At the time of Exubera's discontinuation, several other companies were pursuing inhaled insulin including Alkermes working with Eli Lilly and Company, MannKind Corporation, and Aradigm working with Novo Nordisk.

By March 2008, all of these products had been discontinued except for MannKind's Afrezza product.

On March 16, 2009 MannKind submitted an NDA for their inhalable insulin. In 2011 the FDA denied approval of Afrezza and requested additional clinical trials to its product, the design of which had changed, to ensure that people would use it the same way as the earlier versions.

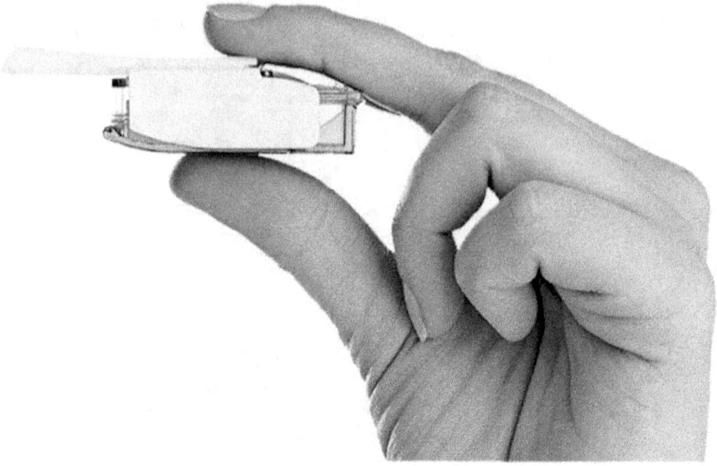

Photo credit: Afrezza/Mannkind

After conducting further studies, Mannkind submitted a new application, and in June, 2014, the FDA approved Afrezza for both Type 1 and Type 2 adult diabetics, with a label restriction for patients having asthma, active lung cancer or COPD.

Landmark discoveries

- ✓ Discovery of insulin by Dr. Frederick Banting in 1921.
- ✓ The distinction between what is now known as Type 1 Diabetes and Type 2 Diabetes was first clearly made by Sir Harold Percival *(Harry)* Himsworth, and published in January 1936.
- ✓ Development of the long acting insulin NPH in the 1940s by Novo-Nordisk
- ✓ Identification of the first of the sulfonylureas in 1942
- ✓ Reintroduction of the use of biguanides for Type 2 Diabetes in the late 1950s. The initial phenformin was withdrawn worldwide *(in the U.S. in 1977)* due to its potential for sometimes fatal lactic acidosis and metformin was first marketed in France in 1979, but not until 1994 in the US.
- ✓ The determination of the amino acid sequence of insulin by Sir Frederick Sanger, for which he received a Nobel Prize. Insulin was the first protein that the amino acid structure was determined.
- ✓ The radioimmunoassay for insulin, as discovered by Rosalyn Yalow and Solomon Berson *(gaining Yalow the 1977 Nobel Prize in Physiology or Medicine)*
- ✓ The three-dimensional structure of insulin *(PDB: 2INS)*
- ✓ Dr Gerald Reaven's identification of the constellation of symptoms now called metabolic syndrome in 1988
- ✓ Demonstration that intensive glycemic control in Type 1 Diabetes reduces chronic side effects more as glucose levels approach "*normal*" in a large longitudinal study, and also in Type 2 Diabetics in other large studies
- ✓ Identification of the first thiazolidinedione as an effective insulin sensitizer during the 1990s
- ✓ In 1980, U.S. biotech company Genentech developed biosynthetic human insulin. The insulin was isolated from genetically altered bacteria *(the bacteria contain the human gene for synthesizing synthetic human insulin)*, which produce large quantities of insulin.

The purified insulin is distributed to pharmacies for use by Diabetes patients. Initially, this development was not regarded by the medical profession as a clinically meaningful development. However, by 1996, the advent of insulin analogues which had vastly improved absorption, distribution, metabolism, and excretion *(ADME)* characteristics which were clinically meaningful based on this early biotechnology development.

Managing Diabetes

"MEASURING THE BLOOD SUGAR LEVEL IS ALWAYS CRITICAL"

People with Diabetes can live long and healthy lives if their Diabetes is detected and well-managed. Facilities for Diabetes diagnosis and management should be available in primary health-care settings, with an established referral and back-referral system.

Good management, using a standardized protocol can potentially prevent complications and premature death from Diabetes using: a small set of generic medicines, interventions to promote healthy lifestyles, patient education to facilitate self-care, regular screening for early detection and treatment of complications through a multidisciplinary team.

Although before we treat our Diabetes we have multiple solutions for the optional approach such as non-invasive measurement tools on skin, eyes, ears, stomach. Also it is very important to understand that in some cases our body is capable to fight with the Diabetes by changing our lifestyle. This is especially true for Type 2 Diabetes and Gestational Diabetes.

But we should not mix this with Type 1 Diabetes because people with Type 1 Diabetes always need to use insulin. While Type 2 Diabetes might be treatable even without serious medications. Also in case a medication is needed there are many oral medications helping the Type 2 patients.

The dark side of using insulin treatment that it can lead any Diabetes patent to low blood sugar *(Hypoglycemia)*, less than 70 mg/dl *(3.9 mmol/l)*. Hypoglycemia is a very common occurrence in people with Diabetes, usually the result of a mismatch in the balance among insulin, food and physical activity.

Mild cases are self-treated by eating or drinking something high in sugar.

Severe cases can lead to unconsciousness and are treated with intravenous glucose or injections with glucagon.

Measuring the blood sugar level is always critical. Continuous glucose monitors can alert patients to the presence of dangerously high or low blood sugar levels.

If the blood sugar level is not well controlled, may cause blindness, kidney failure, lower limb amputation and several other serious long-term complications that impact significantly on quality of life. Furthermore, complications may arise from low blood sugar caused by excessive insulin treatment.

There are no global estimates of Diabetes-related end-stage renal disease, cardiovascular events, lower-extremity amputations or pregnancy complications, though these conditions affect many people living with Diabetes. Where data are available – mostly from high-income countries – prevalence, incidence and trends vary hugely between countries.

Controlling blood glucose levels and cardiovascular disease risk through counseling to promote a healthy diet and physical activity, and through use of medicines, is considered a *"best buy"* for reducing the health impact.

Hypoglycemia

Hypoglycemia, also known as low blood sugar or low blood glucose. We are talking about Hypoglycemia when the blood sugar decreases to below normal levels.

This may result in a variety of symptoms including clumsiness, trouble talking, confusion, loss of consciousness, seizures, or death. A feeling of hunger, sweating, shakiness, and weakness may also be present. Symptoms typically come on quickly.

The most common cause of Hypoglycemia is medications used to treat Diabetes Mellitus such as insulin, sulfonylureas, and biguanides. Risk is greater in diabetics who have eaten less than usual, exercised more than usual, or have drunk alcohol.

Other causes of Hypoglycemia include kidney failure, certain tumors, liver disease, hypothyroidism, starvation, inborn error of metabolism, severe infections, reactive Hypoglycemia, and a number of drugs including alcohol.

Low blood sugar may occur in babies who are otherwise healthy who have not eaten for a few hours.

The glucose level that defines Hypoglycemia is variable. In **people with Diabetes** levels **below 3.9 mmol/L** *(70 mg/dL)* is diagnostic.

In **adults without Diabetes**, symptoms related to low blood sugar, low blood sugar at the time of symptoms, and improvement when blood sugar is restored to normal confirm the diagnosis. Otherwise a level **below 2.8 mmol/L** *(50 mg/dL)* after not eating or following exercise may be used.

In **newborns** a level **below 2.2 mmol/L** *(40 mg/dL)* or less than 3.3 mmol/L (*60 mg/dL*) if symptoms are present indicates Hypoglycemia.

Hypoglycemic **symptoms and manifestations** can be divided into those produced by the counterregulatory hormones *(epinephrine/adrenaline and glucagon)* triggered by the falling glucose, and the neuroglycopenic effects produced by the reduced brain sugar.

- Shakiness, anxiety, nervousness
- Palpitations, tachycardia
- Sweating, feeling of warmth *(sympathetic muscarinic rather than adrenergic)*
- Pallor, coldness, clamminess
- Dilated pupils *(mydriasis)*
- Hunger, borborygmus
- Nausea, vomiting, abdominal discomfort
- Headache

Among people with Diabetes, **prevention** is by matching the foods eaten, with the amount of exercise, and the medications used. When people feel their blood sugar is low testing with a glucose monitor is recommended.

Some people have few initial symptoms of low blood sugar and frequent routine testing in this group is recommended.

Other signs of the Hypoglycemia in the Central nervous system:

- Abnormal thinking, impaired judgment
- Nonspecific dysphoria, moodiness, depression, crying, exaggerated concerns
- Feeling of numbness, pins and needles *(paresthesia)*
- Negativism, irritability, belligerence, combativeness, rage
- Personality change, emotional lability
- Fatigue, weakness, apathy, lethargy, daydreaming, sleep
- Confusion, memory loss, lightheadedness or dizziness, delirium
- Staring, glassy look, blurred vision, double vision
- Flashes of light in the field of vision
- Automatic behavior, also known as automatism
- Difficulty speaking, slurred speech
- Ataxia, incoordination, sometimes mistaken for drunkenness

- ➡ Focal or general motor deficit, paralysis, hemiparesis
- ➡ Headache
- ➡ Stupor, coma, abnormal breathing
- ➡ Generalized or focal seizures

Not all of the above manifestations occur in every case of Hypoglycemia. There is no consistent order to the appearance of the symptoms, if symptoms even occur. Specific manifestations may also vary by age, by severity of the Hypoglycemia and the speed of the decline.

In young children, vomiting can sometimes accompany morning hypoglycemia with ketosis. In older children and adults, moderately severe Hypoglycemia can resemble mania, mental illness, drug intoxication, or drunkenness.

In the elderly, Hypoglycemia can produce focal stroke-like effects or a hard-to-define malaise. The symptoms of a single person may be similar from episode to episode, but are not necessarily so and may be influenced by the speed at which glucose levels are dropping, as well as previous incidents.

It is also very important to know that a person with Diabetes going through Hypoglycemia can be seen very similar as a drunk one or a drug addict even if he/she has zero narcotics or alcohol in his/her body. In some horrifying stories we often hear Diabetic people leaved behind without any help because of this misbelief.

In newborns, hypoglycemia can produce irritability, jitters, myoclonic jerks, cyanosis, respiratory distress, apneic episodes, sweating, hypothermia, somnolence, hypotonia, refusal to feed, and seizures or "*spells*". Hypoglycemia can resemble asphyxia, hypocalcemia, sepsis, or heart failure.

In both young and old patients, the brain may habituate to low glucose levels, with a reduction of noticeable symptoms despite neuroglycopenic impairment.

In insulin-dependent diabetic patients this phenomenon is termed Hypoglycemia unawareness and is a significant clinical problem when improved glycemic control is attempted.

Another aspect of this phenomenon occurs in Type I glycogenosis, when chronic Hypoglycemia before diagnosis may be better tolerated than acute Hypoglycemia after treatment is underway.

Hypoglycemic symptoms can also occur when one is sleeping. Examples of symptoms during sleep can include damp bed sheets or clothes from perspiration.

Having nightmares or the act of crying out can be a sign of Hypoglycemia. Once the individual is awake they may feel tired, irritable, or confused and these may be signs of Hypoglycemia as well.

In nearly all cases, Hypoglycemia that is severe enough to cause **seizures or unconsciousness can be reversed without obvious harm to the brain**.

Cases of death or permanent neurological damage occurring with a single episode have usually involved prolonged, untreated unconsciousness, interference with breathing, severe concurrent disease, or some other type of vulnerability. Nevertheless, brain damage or death has occasionally resulted from severe Hypoglycemia.

Treatment of Hypoglycemia is by eating foods high in simple sugars or taking dextrose. If a person is not able to take food by mouth, an injection of glucagon may help. The treatment of hypoglycemia unrelated to Diabetes include treating the underlying problem.

Hypoglycemia due to dumping syndrome and other post-surgical conditions is best dealt with by altering diet. Including fat and protein with carbohydrates may slow digestion and reduce early insulin secretion. Some forms of this respond to treatment with a glucosidase inhibitor, which slows starch digestion.

The term "*Hypoglycemia*" is sometimes incorrectly used to refer to idiopathic postprandial syndrome, a controversial condition with similar symptoms that occur following eating but with normal blood sugar levels.

Hyperglycemia

Hyperglycemia, or high blood sugar *(also spelled Hyperglycaemia or Hyperglycæmia, not to be confused with the opposite disorder, Hypoglycemia)* is a condition in which an excessive amount of glucose circulates in the blood plasma.

We are talking about Hyperglycemia in general when the blood sugar level higher than 11.1 mmol/l *(200 mg/dl)*, but symptoms may not start to become noticeable until even higher values such as 15–20 mmol/l *(~250–300 mg/dl)*.

The origin of the term is Greek: prefix ὑπέρ- hyper- *("over-")*, γλυκός glycos *("sweet wine, must")*, αἷμα haima *("blood")*, -ία, -εια -ia suffix for abstract nouns of feminine gender.

It is critical for patients to continuously measure the blood sugar level, since chronic levels exceeding 7 mmol/l *(125 mg/dl)* can produce organ damage.

Temporary Hyperglycemia is often benign and asymptomatic. Blood glucose levels can rise well above normal for significant periods without producing any permanent effects or symptoms.

However, chronic Hyperglycemia at levels more than slightly above normal can produce a very wide variety of serious complications over a period of years, including kidney damage, neurological damage, cardiovascular damage, damage to the retina or damage to feet and legs.

Diabetic neuropathy may be a result of long-term hyperglycemia.

In Diabetes Mellitus *(by far the most common cause of chronic Hyperglycemia)* treatment aims at maintaining blood glucose at a level as close to normal as possible, in order to avoid these serious long-term complications. This is done by a combination of proper diet, regular exercise, and insulin or other medication such as Metformin, etc.

Acute hyperglycemia involving glucose levels that are extremely high is a medical emergency and can rapidly produce serious complications *(such as fluid loss through osmotic diuresis)*. It is most often seen in persons who have uncontrolled insulin-dependent Diabetes.

> ***Facts & Myths** Nr 10.*
>
> *Myth:* If you have Diabetes you cannot eat chocolates or sweets
>
> *Fact:* People with Diabetes can eat chocolates and sweets if they combine them with exercise or eat them as part of a healthy meal.

The following symptoms may be associated with acute or chronic Hyperglycemia, with the first three composing the classic hyperglycemic triad:

- ➡ Polyphagia - frequent hunger, especially pronounced hunger
- ➡ Polydipsia - frequent thirst, especially excessive thirst
- ➡ Polyuria - increased volume of urination *(not an increased frequency for urination)*
- ➡ Blurred vision
- ➡ Fatigue
- ➡ Weight loss
- ➡ Poor wound healing *(cuts, scrapes, etc.)*
- ➡ Dry mouth
- ➡ Dry or itchy skin
- ➡ Tingling in feet or heels
- ➡ Erectile dysfunction
- ➡ Recurrent infections, external ear infections *(swimmer's ear)*
- ➡ Cardiac arrhythmia
- ➡ Stupor
- ➡ Coma
- ➡ Seizures

Frequent hunger without other symptoms can also indicate that blood sugar levels are too low. This may occur when people who have Diabetes take too much oral Hypoglycemic medication or insulin for the amount of food they eat.

The resulting drop in blood sugar level to below the normal range prompts a hunger response. This hunger is not usually as pronounced as in Type 1 Diabetes, especially the juvenile onset form, but it makes the prescription of oral hypoglycemic medication difficult to manage.

Polydipsia and polyuria occur when blood glucose levels rise high enough to result in excretion of excess glucose via the kidneys, which leads to the presence of glucose in the urine. This produces an osmotic diuresis.

Hyperglycemia can be a serious problem if not treated in time. In untreated hyperglycemia, a condition called Ketoacidosis *(contrast ketosis)* could occur.

Ketoacidosis develops when the body does not have enough insulin. Without insulin, the body isn't able to utilize the glucose for fuel, so the body starts to break down fats for energy.

The following conditions can also cause hyperglycemia in the absence of Diabetes.

- ➡ Dysfunction of the thyroid, adrenal, and pituitary glands
- ➡ Numerous diseases of the pancreas
- ➡ Severe increases in blood glucose may be seen in sepsis and certain infections
- ➡ Intracranial diseases *(frequently overlooked)* can also cause hyperglycemia. Encephalitis, brain tumors *(especially those located near the pituitary gland)*, brain bleeds, and meningitis are prime examples.
- ➡ Mild to high blood sugar levels are often seen in convulsions and terminal stages of many diseases. Prolonged, major surgeries can temporarily increase glucose levels.
- ➡ Certain forms of severe stress and physical trauma can increase levels for a brief time as well yet rarely exceeds 6.6 mmol/l *(120 mg/dl)*.

A high proportion of patients suffering an **acute stress** such as stroke or myocardial infarction may develop hyperglycemia, even in the absence of a diagnosis of Diabetes. *(Or perhaps stroke or myocardial infarction was caused by hyperglycemia and undiagnosed Diabetes.)* Human and animal studies suggest that this is not benign, and that stress-induced hyperglycemia is associated with a high risk of mortality after both stroke and myocardial infarction.

Exercise related hyperglycemia is caused when hormones *(such as adrenaline and cortisol)* are released during moderate to strenuous exercise. This happens when the muscles signal the liver to release glucose into the bloodstream by converting stored glycogen into glucose.

The cause of exercise related Hypoglycemia, on the other hand, occurs when the muscle group being exercised uses up glucose faster than it can be replenished by the body.

Hyperosmolar Hyperglycemic State

Hyperosmolar Hyperglycemic State *(HHS)* is predominantly a complication of Type 2 Diabetes in which high blood sugars cause severe dehydration, increases in osmolarity (*relative concentration of solute*) and a high risk of complications, coma and death.

Older names for Hyperosmolar Hyperglycemic State are Hyperosmolar Hyperglycemic Nonketotic Coma *(HHNC)*, Hyperosmolar Non-Ketotic Coma *(HONK)*, Nonketotic Hyperosmolar Coma, Hyperosmolar Hyperglycemic Nonketotic Syndrome *(HHNS, favoured by the American Diabetes Association)*.

Hyperosmolar Hyperglycemic State is related to Diabetic Ketoacidosis *(DKA)*, another complication of Diabetes more often encountered in people with Type 1 Diabetes.

In Hyperosmolar Hyperglycemic State the serum **glucose levels** are extremely high, usually **greater than 40-50 mmol/L**, but an anion-gap metabolic acidosis is absent or mild.

It is diagnosed with blood tests and they are differentiated with measurement of ketone bodies, organic molecules that are the underlying driver for Diabetic Ketoacidosis but are usually not detectable in Hyperosmolar Hyperglycemic State.

According to the consensus statement published by the American Diabetes Association, diagnostic features of Hyperosmolar Hyperglycemic State may include the following:

- Plasma glucose level >600 mg/dL *(>30 mmol/L)*
- Serum osmolality >320 mOsm/kg
- Profound dehydration, up to an average of 9L *(and therefore substantial thirst (polydipsia))*
- Serum pH >7.30
- Bicarbonate >15 mEq/L
- Small ketonuria *(~+ on dipstick)* and absent-to-low ketonemia *(<3 mmol/L)*
- Some alteration in consciousness

Additionally it may also lead to:

- Neurologic signs including focal signs such as sensory or motor impairments or focal seizures or motor abnormalities, including flaccidity, depressed reflexes, tremors or fasciculations.
- Hyperviscosity and increased risk of blood clot formation

Nonketotic coma is usually precipitated by an infection, myocardial infarction, stroke or another acute illness. A relative insulin deficiency leads to a serum glucose that is usually higher than 33 mmol/L *(600 mg/dL)*, and a resulting serum osmolarity that is greater than 320 mOsm.

This leads to excessive urination *(more specifically an osmotic diuresis)* which in turn leads to volume depletion and hemoconcentration that causes a further increase in blood glucose level. Ketosis is absent because the presence of some insulin inhibits hormone-sensitive lipase mediated fat tissue breakdown.

The **treatment** of Hyperosmolar Hyperglycemic State consists of correction of the dehydration with intravenous fluids, reestablishing tissue perfusion, reduction of the blood sugar levels with insulin, and management of any underlying conditions that might have precipitated the illness, such as an acute infection.

Diabetic ketoacidosis

Diabetic Ketoacidosis *(DKA)* happens predominantly in those with Type 1 Diabetes and it is a potentially life-threatening complication in people with Diabetes Mellitus. Under certain circumstances Diabetic Ketoacidosis can occur in those with Type 2 Diabetes as well.

Without treatment Diabetic Ketoacidosis can lead to death. Diabetic Ketoacidosis occurs in 0.46% – 0.8% of people with Type 1 Diabetes annually.

It was first described in 1886 and until the introduction of insulin therapy in the 1920s, it was almost universally fatal. It now carries a mortality of less than 1% with adequate and timely treatment.

The first full description of Diabetic Ketoacidosis is attributed to Julius Dreschfeld, a German pathologist working in Manchester, United Kingdom. In his description which he gave in an 1886 lecture at the Royal College of Physicians in London, he drew on reports by Adolph Kussmaul as well as describing the main ketones, acetoacetate and β-hydroxybutyrate, and their chemical determination.

Diabetic Ketoacidosis results from a shortage of insulin; in response the body switches to burning fatty acids and producing acidic ketone bodies that cause most of the symptoms and complications. Diabetic Ketoacidosis may be the first symptom of previously undiagnosed Diabetes, but it may also occur in people known to have Diabetes as a result of a variety of causes, such as intercurrent illness or poor compliance with insulin therapy.

Signs and symptoms of Diabetic Ketoacidosis may include:

➡ Ketoacidosis

➡ Kussmaul hyperventilation: deep, rapid breathing

➡ Confusion or a decreased level of consciousness

➡ Dehydration due to glycosuria and osmotic diuresis

➡ Acute hunger and/or thirst

- ➡ 'Fruity' smelling breath odor
- ➡ Impairment of cognitive function, along with increased sadness and anxiety

The **symptoms** of an episode of Diabetic Ketoacidosis usually evolve over the period of about 24 hours. Predominant symptoms are nausea and vomiting, pronounced thirst, excessive urine production and abdominal pain that may be severe. Those who measure their glucose levels themselves may notice Hyperglycemia *(high blood sugar levels)*.

In severe Diabetic Ketoacidosis, breathing becomes labored and of a deep, gasping character *(a state referred to as "Kussmaul respiration")*. The abdomen may be tender to the point that an acute abdomen may be suspected, such as acute pancreatitis, appendicitis or gastrointestinal perforation.

Coffee ground vomiting *(vomiting of altered blood)* occurs in a minority of people; this tends to originate from erosion of the esophagus. In severe Diabetic Ketoacidosis there may be confusion, lethargy, stupor or even coma *(a marked decrease in the level of consciousness)*.

About **30% of children with Type 1 Diabetes** receive their diagnosis after an episode of Diabetic Ketoacidosis.

Small children with Diabetic Ketoacidosis are relatively prone to cerebral edema *(swelling of the brain tissue)*, which may cause headache, coma, loss of the pupillary light reflex, and progress to death.

It occurs in 0.3–1.0% of children with Diabetic Ketoacidosis, and has been described in young adults, but is overall very rare in adults. It carries a 20–50% mortality.

Young people with recurrent episodes of Diabetic Ketoacidosis may have an underlying eating disorder, or may be using insufficient insulin for fear that it will cause weight gain.

On physical examination there is usually clinical evidence of dehydration, such as a dry mouth and decreased skin turgor. If the dehydration is profound enough to cause a decrease in the circulating blood volume, tachycardia *(a fast heart rate)* and low blood pressure may be observed.

Often, a "*ketotic*" odor is present, which is often described as "*fruity*", often compared to the smell of pear drops whose scent is a ketone. If Kussmaul respiration is present, this is reflected in an increased respiratory rate.

Treatment involves intravenous fluids to correct dehydration, insulin to suppress the production of ketone bodies, treatment for any underlying causes such as infections, and close observation to prevent and identify complications.

Diabetic Ketoacidosis arises because of a lack of insulin in the body. The lack of insulin and corresponding elevation of glucagon leads to increased release of glucose by the liver *(a process that is normally suppressed by insulin)* from glycogen via glycogenolysis and also through gluconeogenesis.

High glucose levels spill over into the urine, taking water and solutes *(such as sodium and potassium)* along with it in a process known as osmotic diuresis. This leads to polyuria, dehydration, and compensatory thirst and polydipsia.

The absence of insulin also leads to the release of free fatty acids from adipose tissue *(lipolysis)*, which are converted through a process called beta oxidation, again in the liver, into ketone bodies *(acetoacetate and β-hydroxybutyrate)*.

β-Hydroxybutyrate can serve as an energy source in the absence of insulin-mediated glucose delivery, and is a protective mechanism in case of starvation. The ketone bodies, however, have a low pKa and therefore turn the blood acidic *(metabolic acidosis)*.

The body initially buffers the change with the bicarbonate buffering system, but this system is quickly overwhelmed and other mechanisms must work to compensate for the acidosis.

One such mechanism is hyperventilation to lower the blood carbon dioxide levels *(a form of compensatory respiratory alkalosis)*. This hyperventilation, in its extreme form, may be observed as Kussmaul respiration.

In various situations such as infection, insulin demands rise but are not matched by the failing pancreas. Blood sugars rise, dehydration ensues, and resistance to the normal effects of insulin increases further by way of a vicious circle.

As a result of the above mechanisms, the average adult with Diabetic Ketoacidosis has a total body water shortage of about 6 liters *(or 100 mL/kg)*, in addition to substantial shortages in sodium, potassium, chloride, phosphate, magnesium and calcium. Glucose levels usually exceed 13.8 mmol/L or 250 mg/dL.

If Diabetic Ketoacidosis occurs in someone with Type 2 Diabetes, their condition is called "**Ketosis-Prone Type 2 Diabetes**". The exact mechanism for this phenomenon is unclear, but there is evidence both of impaired insulin secretion and insulin action.

Once the condition has been treated, insulin production resumes and often the person may be able to resume diet or tablet treatment as normally recommended in Type 2 Diabetes.

The entity of Ketosis-Prone Type 2 Diabetes was first fully described in 1987 after several preceding case reports.

It was initially thought to be a form of maturity onset Diabetes of the young, and went through several other descriptive names *(such as "Idiopathic Type 1 Diabetes", "Flatbush Diabetes", "Atypical Diabetes" and "Type 1.5 Diabetes")* before the current terminology of "Ketosis-Prone Type 2 Diabetes" was adopted.

Attacks of Diabetic Ketoacidosis can be **prevented** in those known to have Diabetes to an extent by adherence to "*sick day rules*". These are clear-cut instructions to person on how to treat themselves when unwell. Instructions include advice on how much extra insulin to take when sugar levels appear uncontrolled, an easily digestible diet rich in salt and carbohydrates, means to suppress fever and treat infection, and recommendations when to call for medical help.

The main aims in the **treatment of Diabetic Ketoacidosis** are replacing the lost fluids and electrolytes while suppressing the high blood sugars and ketone production with insulin. Admission to an intensive care unit or similar high-dependency area or ward for close observation may be necessary.

The amount of fluid replaced depends on the estimated degree of dehydration. If dehydration is so severe as to cause shock *(severely decreased blood pressure with insufficient blood supply to the body's organs)*, or a depressed level of consciousness, rapid infusion of saline *(1 liter for adults, 10 ml/kg in repeated doses for children)* is recommended to restore circulating volume.

Slower rehydration based on calculated water and sodium shortage may be possible if the dehydration is moderate, and again saline is the recommended fluid.

Very mild Ketoacidosis with no associated vomiting and mild dehydration may be treated with oral rehydration and subcutaneous rather than intravenous insulin under observation for signs of deterioration.

A special but unusual consideration is cardiogenic shock, where the blood pressure is decreased not due to dehydration but due to inability of the heart to pump blood through the blood vessels.

This situation requires ICU admission, monitoring of the central venous pressure *(which requires the insertion of a central venous catheter in a large upper body vein)*, and the administration of medication that increases the heart pumping action and blood pressure.

The administration of sodium bicarbonate solution to rapidly improve the acid levels in the blood is controversial.

There is little evidence that it improves outcomes beyond standard therapy, and indeed some evidence that while it may improve the acidity of the blood, it may actually worsen acidity inside the body's cells and increase the risk of certain complications. Its use is therefore discouraged, although some guidelines recommend it for extreme acidosis *(pH<6.9)*, and smaller amounts for severe acidosis *(pH 6.9–7.0)*.

Brittle Diabetes

"*Brittle*" Diabetes, also known as Unstable Diabetes or Labile Diabetes, is a term that was traditionally used to describe the dramatic and recurrent swings in glucose levels, often occurring for no apparent reason in insulin-dependent Diabetes.

The results of such swings can be accompanied by irregular and unpredictable high blood sugar levels, frequently with ketosis, and sometimes with serious low blood sugar levels.

An insulin pump may be recommended for brittle Diabetes to reduce the number of Hypoglycemic episodes and better control the morning rise of blood sugar due to the dawn phenomenon.

Because labile Diabetes is defined as

> "*episodes of Hypoglycemia or Hyperglycemia that, whatever their cause, constantly disrupt a patient's life*",

it can have many causes, some of which include:

- ➡ errors in Diabetes management which can include too much insulin being given in ratio to carbohydrate being consumed
- ➡ interactions with other medical conditions
- ➡ psychological problems
- ➡ biological factors that interfere with how insulin is processed within the body
- ➡ Hypoglycemia and Hyperglycemia due to strenuous exercise, however Hypoglycemia is more frequent
- ➡ insulin exposed to higher temperatures that reduces effectiveness of the insulin hormone in the body
- ➡ spontaneous production of insulin in the body due to activity in the beta cells during the period shortly after diagnosis of Type 1 Diabetes

Brittle Diabetes occurs no more frequently than in 1% to 2% of Diabetics and some experts even say the "*brittle Diabetes*" concept "*has no biologic basis and should not be used*".

In a small study, 10 of 20 brittle diabetic patients aged 18–23 years who could be traced had died within 22 years, and the remainder, though suffering high rates of complications, were no longer brittle. These results were similar to those of an earlier study by the same authors which found a 19% mortality in 26 patients after 10.5 years.

Measuring the blood sugar

Continuous blood sugar level monitoring is the part of the daily routine of the Diabetic people.

It is critical for patients who monitor glucose levels at home to be aware of which units of measurement their testing kit uses.

Glucose levels are measured in either:

- Millimoles per liter *(mmol/l)* is the **SI standard** unit used in most countries around the world.
- Milligrams per deciliter *(mg/dl)* is used in some countries such as the United States, Japan, France, Egypt and Colombia.
- Scientific journals are moving towards using mmol/l, some journals now use mmol/l as the primary unit but quote mg/dl in parentheses.

Normal blood sugar level

The normal blood sugar level for Diabetics should be always

between 4,5 mmol/l and 7,7 mmol/l.

(between 80 mg/dl and 140 mg/dl)

Diabetes management can be strengthened through implementation of standards and protocols, even in low-resource settings.

It is highly recommended to create and manage a spreadsheet where all the measurement results can be administrated.

Recommended **measurement** periods are **7 times a day**:

- ➡ Before breakfast
- ➡ 2 hours after breakfast
- ➡ Before lunch
- ➡ 2 hours after lunch
- ➡ Before dinner
- ➡ 2 hours after dinner
- ➡ Before sleeping

Additional data for the better understanding of the body reaction:

- ➡ Time *(hour and minute)*
- ➡ Size of the meal *(Half, Small, Big)*
- ➡ Your mood on a scale of:
  1 (bad/weak) - 2 - 3 - 4 - 5 (perfect, fit)
- ➡ Amount of insulin injected

From these basic information your Diabetes advisor and doctor can gain useful information.

All these data can used as a trend graph showing the time periods, mood situations where an additional correction in the medications, insulin quantity or in the meal plan might be requested.

Glucose levels vary before and after meals, and at various times of day; the definition of "*normal*" varies among medical professionals.

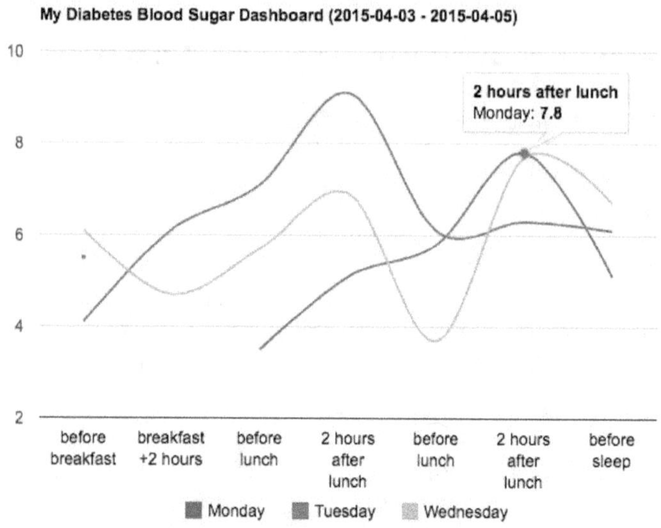

Photo credit: Sugar Guard/Diabetes-Cure.me

A person with a consistent range above 7 mmol/l or 126 mg/dl is generally held to have Hyperglycemia, whereas a consistent range below 4 mmol/l or 70 mg/dl is considered Hypoglycemic. In fasting adults, blood plasma glucose should not exceed 7 mmol/l or 126 mg/dL.

Sustained higher levels of blood sugar cause damage to the blood vessels and to the organs they supply, leading to the complications of Diabetes.

Insulin treatment

People with Type 1 Diabetes require continuous insulin injection for survival. For all the other Diabetic people there are various oral agents, pills and drugs that can help to reduce the blood sugar. In many cases even a change of lifestyle and a new diet can be also effective.

Without insulin, even for a short time *(such as 6 hours)* the Type 1 Diabetic individuals may face life-threatening consequences. Yet an array of international and national barriers interact to hamper access to insulin, and many in low- and middle-income countries do not receive this essential treatment.

The insulin market is dominated by a small number of multinational manufacturers with a few, smaller producers making up only 4% of the market by volume.

This limited competition can potentially increase insulin prices. Additional factors in the insulin market that may impact price include different insulin formulations coming off-patent, as well as the considerable increase in use of analogue insulin. Both of these factors affect the price of insulin before it ever arrives in a given country.

Low-income countries generally pay most for insulin while high and middle-income countries pay least.

The costs associated with diabetes are enormous, it includes expenses related to acute and chronic complications, the costs of therapies to prevent them, and the fact that those affected may be unable to work and support their families. Many patients are pushed into bankruptcy.

People should not be forced into poverty because of the cost of Diabetes care. Remember that Dr. Frederick Banting sold the patent for insulin for one dollar, basically made the insulin patent available without charge and did not attempt to control commercial production.

As the author of present book I have Type 1 Diabetes and I am forced to spend every months almost the half of the minimal wage in Germany for my insulins and my related tools such as needles and blood sugar measurement strips. It is crazy.

Although since I partly live in France as well, I know that the French Government supports the Diabetes medicines and I can refill my monthly supplies for half of the price there. But it is still relatively expensive, but at least we have these supplies in Europe.

> ***Facts & Myths*** *Nr 11.*
>
> *Myth:* I have to go on insulin, this must mean my Diabetes is severe
>
> *Fact:* People take insulin when diet alone or diet with oral or non-insulin injectable Diabetes drugs do not provide good-enough Diabetes control, that's all. Insulin helps Diabetes control. It does not usually have anything to do with the severity of the disease.

Insulin must be injected, meaning syringes are also a survival need for people using insulin. Value added taxes are frequently applied to syringes, which are not readily available in the public sector. If syringes are purchased by the public sector, quantities are often insufficient and not linked to insulin purchases.

Pen injection devices and insulin cartridges have some advantages over traditional syringes *(being more practical when multiple daily injections of insulin are required)* but their cost prohibits their use for many patients.

The lack of access to affordable insulin remains a key impediment to successful treatment and results in needless complications and premature deaths.

Insulin and oral Hypoglycaemic agents are reported as generally available in only a minority of low-income countries. Moreover, essential medicines critical to gaining control of Diabetes, such as agents to lower blood pressure and lipid levels, are frequently unavailable in low- and middle-income countries.

Governments' decisions about insulin purchasing– tendering practices, choice of supplier, choice of products and delivery devices can have a huge impact on budgets and on costs to end users. Governments may recoup high costs by charging mark-ups to patients.

Non-Invasive tools

There are multiple, existing technologies to make the blood sugar measurement more comfortable for people living with Diabetes.

Instead of the often painful finger pricking which means using needle to draw blood from our fingertip, there are possibilities to measure blood sugar level on many other surfaces of our body, such as the eyes, ears, surface of the skin, sweat, tissue fluid, without involving any blood.

These new non-invasive, 100% pain-free tools and devices makes traditional blood sampling a thing of the past, allowing you to monitor blood glucose levels without the need to pierce your skin.

There are many situations whereby conventional testing is challenging. Surveys show that over 90% of people with Diabetes would welcome a continuous blood glucose monitoring solution whilst driving and during sports or other physical activity.

Also 56% of people with Diabetes would test themselves between 8-10 times per day if testing would be painless, compared to just 18.3% who are already testing themselves that many times.

Not to mention that regular blood sugar testing with the traditional test strips comes with a very high cost, typically exceeding 1.000 Euro *(800 GBP or 1.100 USD)* per year.

These costs often have withholding powers and in low- or middle-income families health becomes a secondary issue because of these financial matters.

So pain and costs of the traditional blood sugar monitoring are key issues, however there are many alternative solutions and some of them already available.

I have been searching for less invasive ways to monitor glucose since many years and in this chapter I am aiming to show you a selected few of these solutions ranging from the contact lens, or Diabetes tattoo or even wearable devices.

What is really important is the fact that the technology is ready to positively change the lives of 422 million people living with Diabetes and this is a game changer.

Not to mention that monitoring glucose in a non-invasive, fashionable way is certainly one of the most important fields in the area of wearable health sensors.

So please find here my collections of Non-Invasive tools. *(I am not in any form of business relation with the following companies, they did not support financially the book. I considered it interesting to introduce their way of approach for a non-invasive blood sugar monitoring.)*

Glucose-Sensing Contact Lens

In 2014 the software giant Google announced its glucose-sensing contact lens specially design and developed for people with Diabetes Mellitus.

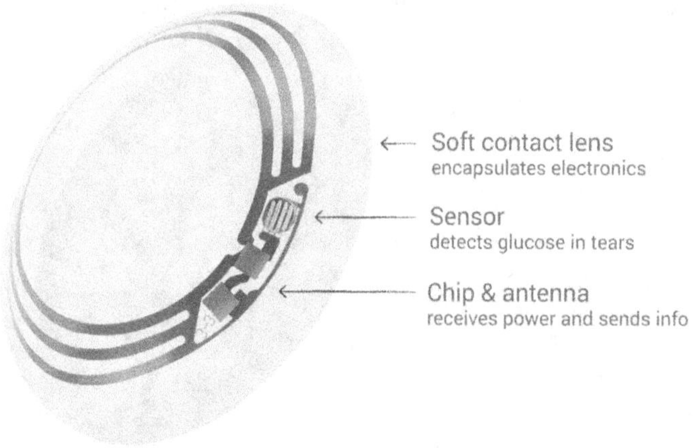

A contact lens with embedded circuitry to monitor blood glucose levels

Photo credit: Google

The system would likely contain two or three parts:

1. the contact lens itself, which would sense glucose levels;
2. a "*reader*" device, which would communicate and power the contact lens; and
3. a user display, which would allow patients to see and review the data. The reader and user display could be on the same device.

In March 2015 Google already received their patent for the Glucose-Sensing Contact Lens.

The patent specifically mentions the possibility of eyeglasses, jewelry *(e.g., earrings, necklace)*, or clothing *(e.g., a scarf, hat, headband)* functioning as the reader.

The main requirement is that the device must be close enough to one of the lenses to make sure that the lens can communicate with the reader, which gives Google a lot of flexibility to be creative!

Similarly, the display device could be a smart phone or wearable computer. One example given is a display worn on the head or in front of the eyes, such as Google Glass *(another project in the Google[x] division)*.

The patent describes how high and low alarms might work and how continuous data could be displayed, suggesting that Google's ultimate goal may be a CGM-like technology.

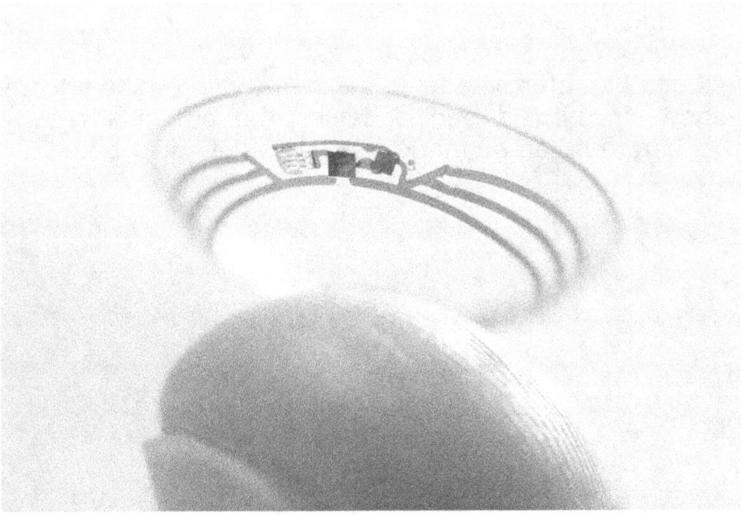

Photo credit: Google

The smart contact lens could be the same size as standard contact lenses and could be made of the same *(or similar)* material. In theory, they might not feel any different to wear than a normal contact lens.

From a convenience perspective alone, a glucose-sensing contact lens powered by clothing/jewelry/glasses could offer a major win for patients, potentially no need to carry around an extra device, significant discretion, and high "*cool factor.*"

Of course, there are still challenges to overcome, such as accuracy and reliability, not to mention cost and manufacturing.

After the first announcement of the Glucose-Sensing Contact Lens by Google, the pharmaceutical giant Novartis partnered up with Google in July 2014 to help make this idea a reality.

The major element of deal was to license the so-called smart lens technology for Alcon, the eye care unit of Novartis.

Since two years now the project is kept quiet. There is no information about the latest timeline on a prototype, and we can just hope that Google is still working on making this idea a reality.

Although and to be fair, the prototype smart contact lens must undergo many rounds of rigorous testing via human clinical trials, before it can be determined if it is accurate, safe, and effective.
In addition, since it is a medical device, the lens must receive FDA approval before it can be marketed and widely distributed.

Diabetes tattoo

Engineers from the University of California, San Diego have developed an ultra-thin temporary tattoo that can painlessly and accurately monitor the glucose levels of Diabetics. This flexible and easy-to-wear temporary tattoo could help Diabetics manage their condition without daily finger pricks.

The flexible device costs just a few cents and lasts for a day at a time, and early tests have shown that it is just as sensitive as a finger-prick test.

But even cooler is the fact that the system works without blood, by extracting and measuring the glucose from the fluid in between skin cells, and could eventually be adapted to detect other important metabolites in the body, or deliver medicine.

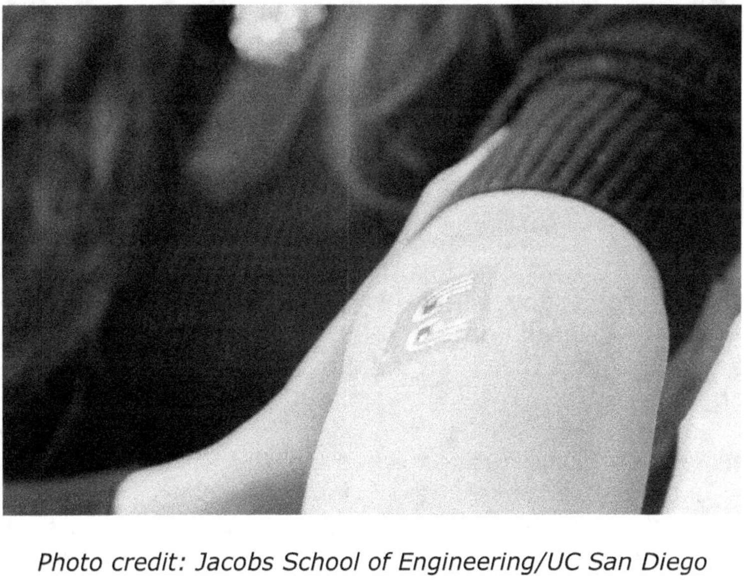

Photo credit: Jacobs School of Engineering/UC San Diego

And the tattoo will allow your blood sugar levels to be continuously measured throughout the day which means to be able to more sensitively maintain the glucose levels and better manage the individual Diabetic conditions.

Created by graduate student Amay Bandodkar, the device is made up of woven electrodes printed out on rub-on tattoo paper, and works by applying a very mild electrical current to the skin for 10 minutes. This forces sodium ions from the fluid between skin cells, which carry glucose, to flow towards the tattoo.

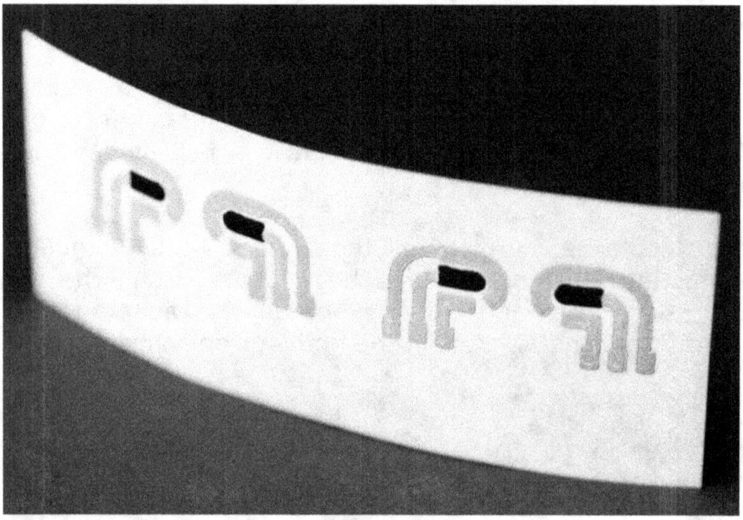

Photo credit: Jacobs School of Engineering/UC San Diego

A sensor built into the tattoo then measures the strength of the electrical charge produced by this glucose. The levels of glucose in this fluid are overall, around 100 times lower than the levels found in someone's blood, so the device requires a more sensitive sensor.

To see how well the tattoo picked up the spike in blood sugar levels expected after a meal, the researchers measured the participants' blood sugar before and after they consumed a carbohydrate-rich sandwich and soda in the lab. The device performed just as well at detecting this glucose spike as a traditional finger-stick monitor, the researchers said.

An early trial on seven men and women aged aged between 20 and 40 without Diabetes has revealed that the users also could not feel anything while wearing the device, other than a mild tingling in the first 10 seconds of use.

The readout instrument will also eventually have Bluetooth capabilities to send this information directly to the patient's doctor in real-time or store data in the cloud.

The scientists are also working on ways to make the tattoo last longer while keeping its overall cost down.

Furthermore the researchers suggested that these devices could also measure other important chemicals such as lactate, which athletes might want to analyze to monitor their fitness, or certain amino acids, which could test how well a medication is working.

Measuring from the Sweat

Already in 2011, the revolutionary concept of bluecircle was born by David Seo. It was design as a bluetooth and usb device to be connected to computers to keep the data organized and updated while it provides a safe and painless method of measuring the glucose levels in the body.

The bluecircle glucose wristband has been designed to monitor the blood glucose level directly from a person's sweat. When a user wearing the band perspires while exercising, the sweat travels through a layer of advanced GSR strip to calculate the blood sugar level ultimately displaying it on the OLED screen.

This non-invasive method thus could help people in knowing their sugar levels before matters get out of hand.

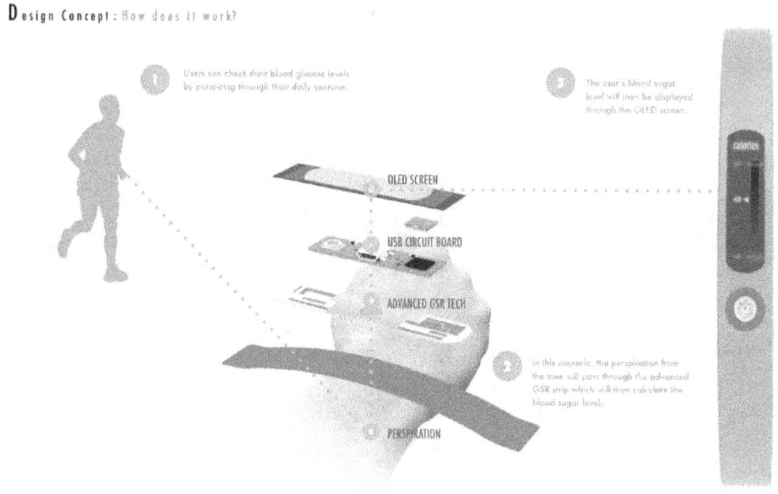

Photo credit: bluecircle by David Seo

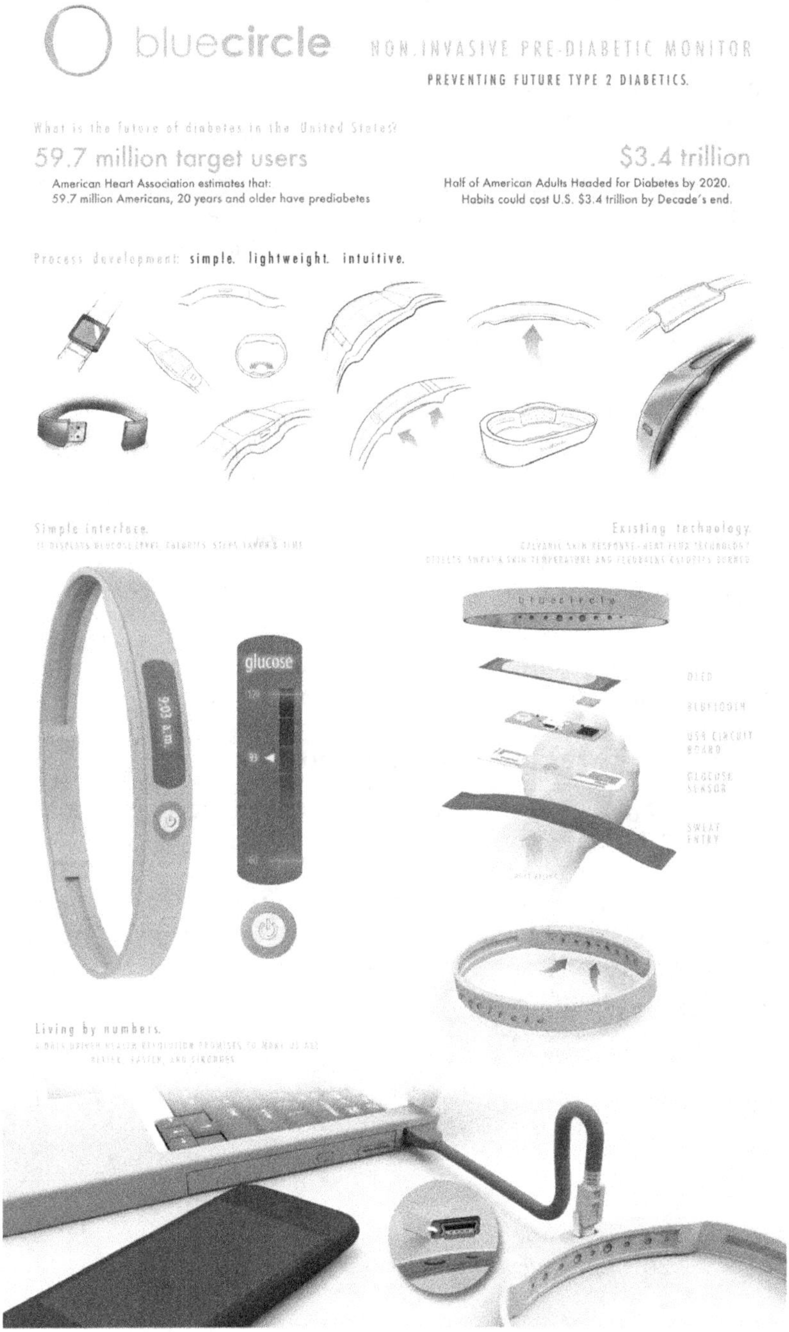

Photo credit: bluecircle by David Seo

Measuring on the Skin

One of the hardest way to measure blood sugar level is through wearable devices on the surface of the skin.

In the human body the skin acts as a barrier to low powered radiation, most of it gets reflected which makes it hard to get good accuracy. Also, skin is very heterogenous, varying a lot from person to person *(race, age, color, atmospheric conditions, etc)*. So non-invasive glucose sensing on the surface of the skin is really hard due to many factors.

This is the main reason that the conventional finger-prick blood glucose monitors have been so dominant in the past 40 years is their ability to provide accurate glucose readings in virtually all humans, independent of their size, age, race or situation they happen to be in. This is because those devices pierce the skin into the blood and at blood level the conditions are much more homogenous.

There are two main approaches for non-invasive glucose monitoring using electromagnetic waves:

- ➡ The first utilizes low-frequency radio waves.
- ➡ The second utilizes much higher frequencies at the optical part of the spectrum.

Unfortunately, none of these methods tackle the problem of bypassing the skin, thus limiting their effectiveness and this is why they need constant recalibration and are only accurate in certain specific conditions.

Few years ago I came across to a solution called GlucoWise. It is a concept for a non-invasive blood sugar sensing tool which I really liked.

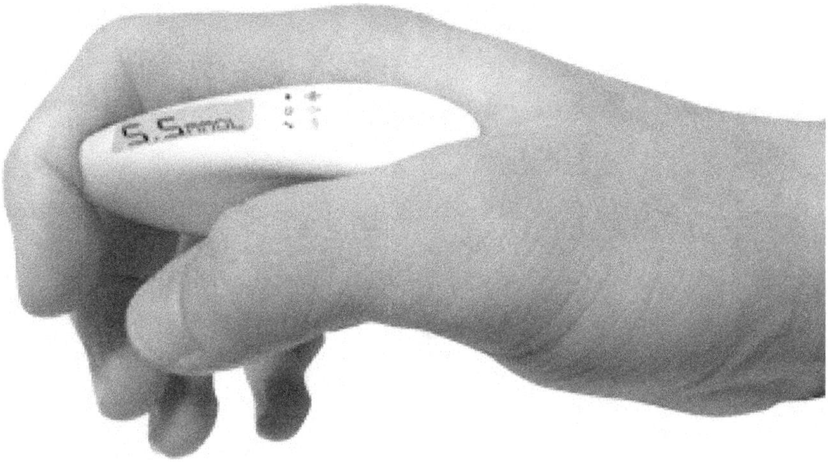

Photo credit: GlucoWise by MediWise

GlucoWise is different because it uses neither optics nor low-frequency microwaves, but rather a "*new*" part of the spectrum between 50 - 100 GHz that has only very recently been technologically available to manipulate, and it utilizes the metamaterial film to bypass the skin problem, providing for the first time person-independent glucose readings.

This non-invasive, wireless device will take an accurate blood glucose reading every few seconds or as often as the user requires. It is positioned to gently squeeze the skin between the thumb and forefinger or the earlobe to measure blood glucose levels. The device then displays the reading in real-time on the screen.

The information collected by the monitor can be also uploaded wirelessly to the mobile app, allowing you to track your readings over time and merge it with other information impacting your blood glucose levels. Data collected will ultimately integrate with other databases, mobile health apps and platforms with the appropriate permissions.

And it is smartly designed because it works effectively in a wide range of climates, humidities and temperatures so you are free to snowboard or jog as much as you please.

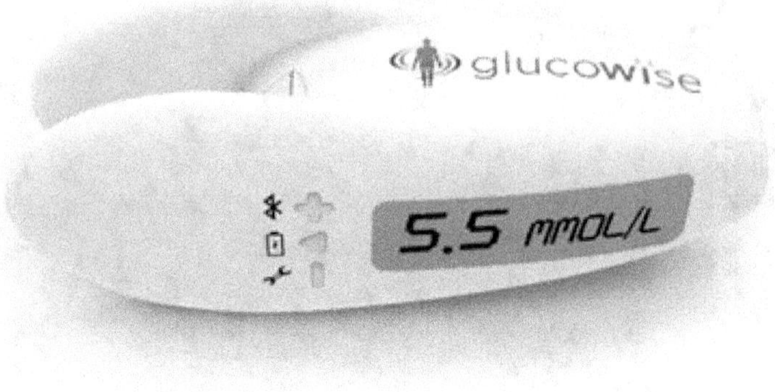

Photo credit: GlucoWise by MediWise

Understanding more about the solutions I believe it has the potential to exceed industry standards for self-monitoring blood glucose accuracy.

The only thing which was painful for me is their planned pricing model. If they get the funds and the FDA approval they would like to charge an almost 15 times higher price to those who suffer from Diabetes than the production price of the devices. This means an over 5.000 USD price tag at the end of the day.

Glucose Monitor Implant

There is another great way for non-invasive blood glucose monitoring with the help of a special implant.

Since 2015, two research labs works jointly to develop a device in the size of a rice grain that can be implanted under the skin and will glow certain colors when fluorescent light is shined upon it.

The colors will correspond to the Diabetics glucose level, allowing an individual to monitor their health without the invasive and sometimes painful procedures available today.

The person using the implant can painlessly and unobtrusively correlate the color changes with their blood sugar level.

The device uses two fluorescent dyes, one is tied to a protein that binds to glucose, and the other is tied to a sugar that competes for the binding site on the protein.

Once it is implemented, doctors allow the skin to heal over it and glucose can be easily and non-invasively monitored for at least three months to a year before it needs replacing.

The project is advancing but it still has some obstacles to overcome, however this would provide a way for diabetics to continuously and non-invasively measure their blood glucose.

Measuring on the Ears

Among the newest innovations there are also blood sugar measuring devices which are measuring directly on the ears.

For example GlucoTrack offers a solution which combines 3 technologies:

- ultrasonic,
- electromagnetic and
- thermal measurements.

GlucoTrack has a very human story. The desire to develop a non-invasive glucose monitor came initially from Integrity co-founder, late Dr. David Freger.

David had Diabetes and like many who suffer from this life-long debilitating disease David was sick and tired of pricking his fingers to draw blood for glucose measurements a few times each day.

Together with two of his trusted colleagues Avner Gal and David Malka, they set out to develop a non-invasive glucose monitor that could provide pain-free measurements.

Following years of intense research and development they determined that the technical challenges of increasing the signal to noise ratio, to obtain a reliable reading without drawing blood, could best be achieved by combining three independent technologies simultaneously.

They developed a proprietary and patented approach of using ultrasound, electromagnetic and thermal measurements with a unique algorithm to weigh each measurement and calculate the weighted average of the three readings.

After short and simple calibration process, there are no test strips required, so there is no additional cost per measurement. No finger pricking, no lancets require when making measurements, needle-free no draw blood involve.

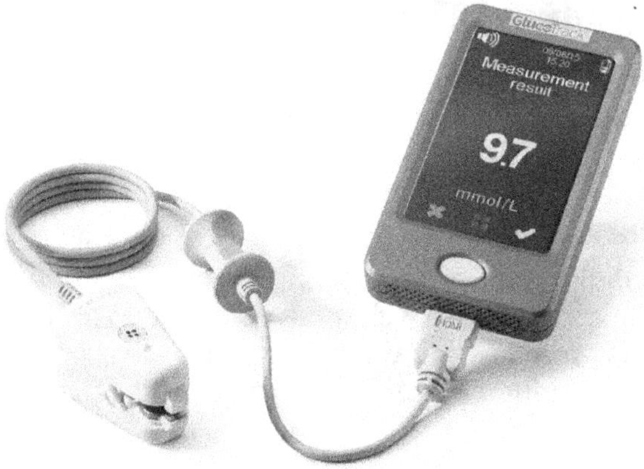

Photo credit: GlucoTrack DF-F by Integrity Applications

It is a highly economic solution due to the fact that you have to replace EarClip only twice a year which offers "*one time*" expense with virtually unlimited measurements.

Sadly Dr. David Freger passed away, however his vision and dedication will always be remembered, this is also reflected by the name choice of the device GlucoTrack model DF-F.

Measuring from the Tissue fluid

"**Diabetes** should not **stand in your way**" says the slogan of MedTronic.

MedTronic offers a highly reliable solutions called MiniMed. It contains an insulin pump with a special sensor. They call it Elite Sensor and it continuously checks your glucose levels, reliably detecting highs and lows. Furthermore the insulin pump is fully integrated with a glucose sensor to give you advanced Diabetes control.

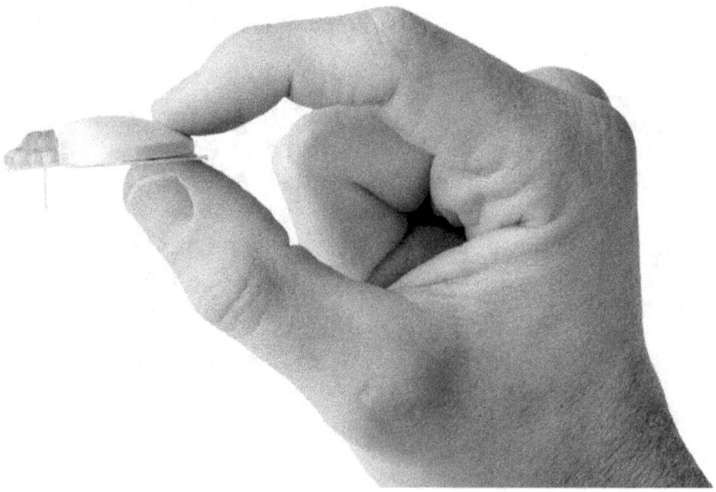

Photo credit: Elite Sensor by MedTronic

This technology helps you to better control your glucose levels and it is the only Diabetes management system which even takes action for you when you need it, so you can be free to experience life's exceptional moments.

Continuous Glucose Monitoring is a great thing which makes it possible for you to see your blood glucose readings in *(almost)* real-time and track historical data.

The problem with the manual blood sugar monitoring is that even if you believe that you know your body, in most cases you are wrong about your blood sugar levels or the perfect timings for the insulin corrections.

It is normal that certain foods and activities are affecting differently our body and to understand these indicators are priceless in your health management. Especially since you can get alerted before the highs and lows happens, so you have a chance to adjust before it is too late.

And to be honest it gives you confidence as well because you do not need to continuously worry about your blood sugar levels.

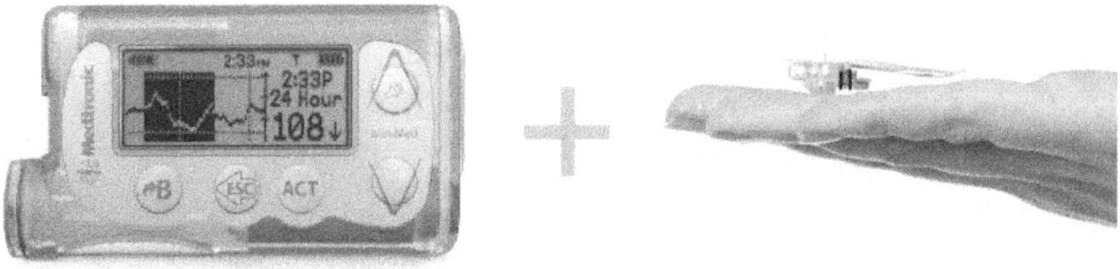

Photo credit: MiniMed & Elite Sensor by MedTronic

How is it work? A tiny electrode called a glucose sensor is inserted under the skin to measure glucose levels in tissue fluid. It is connected to a transmitter that sends the information via wireless radio frequency to a monitoring and display device.

The device can detect and notify you if your glucose is reaching a high or low limit. The latest Medtronic Continuous Glucose Monitoring systems can actually alert you before you reach your glucose limits. It can even take actions for you.

They call it Threshold Suspend. It is a technology that can act for you if your glucose level goes below a preset limit. If you do not respond to alerts, it can pause insulin delivery for up to two hours. You can rest easy, knowing Threshold Suspend is standing guard. It also helps you to exercise and to vary your workout since MiniMed is monitoring your levels as you go.

It's only negative that you have to wear the device all the times, although on the positive side it ensures you a balanced life.

Of course having an insulin pump attached to our body might be more uncomfortable for us adults. Maybe a child can be convinced easier, for example by explaining that he needs it because it gives him super power, just as Tony Stark, the Iron Man has one "*power generator*" in his chest.

From technical point it would not be fair not to mention that the technology is not perfect yet although it is on the market since many years.

The problems is the reliability of the accuracy since the sensor measures your blood sugar level based on the interstitial fluid and not the blood stream. So it can also be outright dangerous if you rely solely on the sensor readings, and ignore what your body is telling you. The funny thing is that you can also read this in the labelling of the Continuous Glucose Monitoring devices, warning you to never adjust insulin based on the sensor reading.

Solutions for Parents and Relatives

Diabetes Mellitus and its different types effect directly Diabetics, although the disease has a great impact on the family and relatives as well.

For example with Type 1, Juvenile Diabetes the parents already have a higher responsibility from the early age of the child. The parents have an obligation to continuously monitor the blood sugar level and to calculate and adjust the insulin based on the daily meals.

Although this process is working well with most of the families at a certain point of life the parents should let their children to kindergarten or school, where they have less control over the environment.

A child with Diabetes always needs support, however among the educators and teachers the willingness to do so is not always there. In fact, kindergartens or schools often refuse to accommodate a child with Diabetes.

Often it is pointed out to parents that one can not assume the responsibility, that the staff is not trained for it and they are fearful to be liable for any errors.

To demonstrate the weight of this problem with an example in Germany there are 17,500 children under 14 years suffering of Diabetes. Up to 2,500 Type 1 Diabetic children added annually, notably children under five. Therefore a very large number of families are struggling to find a kindergarten or a school for their Diabetic children.

And it is an undeniable fact that more and more children get Type 1 Diabetes. This often causes problems for parents in school enrollment or to find a day care place.

Most educators and teachers must be aware that every now and then a child appears with Diabetes in their group or class. They also have to deal with the fact that these children need more attention and help in the management of Diabetes, at least until the end of primary school. It is not so easy, since every child from the age of two has the right to day care or nursery school and the groups are larger.

It is a sad thing, but kindergartens and schools often take a chronically ill child in the class such as a child with asthma over a Diabetic child. Of course there are always exceptions. However a child can not be discriminated under no circumstances just because of an illness.

Sadly families often face with the same problem with elderly homes.

This was also one of my main motivation factor when I initiated the Diabetes-Cure.me project. Already the ability to care for over 422 Million Diabetic people is a game changer. However I wanted to focus also on our next generation, the children who deserve the very best.

The thing is that we are living in a technology driven World. In most of the countries in the World Internet and mobile communication are available. So if technology is granted then it depends only on our willingness whether we offer a medical solution for these Diabetic people which creates a better living quality or not.

Using the Internet of Things technology, there is a possibility to collect information from non-invasive glucose monitoring sensors.

We are capable to ensure children a 100% pain-free Diabetes management device combined with the technological advantage of an analytics and alerting software. This alerting can be a great help for both the educators and the school teachers, and also for the parents and relatives since they can get real-time information about the health and well being of their loved ones.

The maintenance of a solution like this is relatively cheap, since it only requires a WiFi internet router in the kindergarten or the school for the proper data communication.

For the children there are many ways to make the blood glucose monitoring device fun. First of all it can be implemented into any kind of wearables, such as jewelry, watch, bracelet, ear rings, etc. Secondly due to the globally available 3D printing technologies they can customize them. It can be a very fun accessory for the children, while a bullet proof health monitoring tool for the parents and the educators.

Founding Diabetes-cure.me, we decided to offer a solution which puts People into the centre and I believe this is our unique advantage. The unique combination of our Cloud based software platform and the future non-invasive medical device is that it allows people all around the World to be in charge in the fight against the Diabetes disease.

The aim is to have one place to store all the Diabetes treatment related information and it can be also a real-time connection between the patients and the doctors. It also includes wide range of real-time reports to help to track the key health indicators and influencing activities, events.

Once you give permissions, your doctor can see your real-time reports and there are possibilities for suggestions and immediate adjustments in your treatment.

It could be also a global solution for children, elderly people and all those in needs for control over their Diabetic state. A solution which puts People into the centre, which I believe is our unique advantage.

Of course for a solution such as we aim with Diabetes-Cure.me has the same old problem. As a medical device it needs a CE or FDA approval which takes millions of Euros and without a joint common effort the idea will die due to the lack of funds. Although imagine the piece of mind feeling that a solution such as this one could offer for millions of families.

One of the most dangerous time period for people with Diabetes is at night, so now people with Diabetes could have a continuos sugar guard.

Or imagine having a sudden Hypoglycemic event whilst driving or imagine the situation when you accidentally under-dose your child. This solution could alert you and your loved ones, it would be able to send readings back to their mobile app even when they are not present.

Most importantly you could be constantly aware of the health of your loved ones.

Possible cures

"THE SIMPLEST EXPLANATION IS THAT IT IS FAR TOO PROFITABLE TO TREAT DIABETES THAN CURE IT."

Diabetes was the eighth leading cause of death among both sexes and the fifth leading cause of death of women in 2012. *(Latest data available.)*

The total burden of deaths from high blood glucose in 2012 has been estimated to amount to 3.7 million. Also in 2012 there were 1.5 million deaths worldwide directly caused by Diabetes.

It is a deeply tragic statistic and it raises the question where is the cure? Are we even close to it? Or is it already there somewhere hidden?

Well, it is there... Sort of...

The good news for Pre-Diabetic and Type 2 Diabetes patients is that they have the easier way to be cured.

Also for Type 1 Diabetes a variety of immunological approaches have been successful at preventing a disease similar to human Type 1 Diabetes, it is very clear now for researchers what exactly causes Type 1 Diabetes. Not to mention that surgical ways such as implementing a secondary pancreas can offer full and quality life.

Not all tpossibilities are recommended to everyone, however we have to note that there are multiple options. Options which are rarely talked out publicly, even more the promise of the cure is mystified. For this reason many people believe that a cure might never happen.

The simplest explanation is that it is far too profitable to treat the Diabetes than cure it.

The largest number of deaths resulting from high blood glucose occur in upper-middle income countries *(1.5 million)* and the lowest number in low-income countries *(0.3 million)*. And even if there is a business potential to sell high priced cure drugs to these upper-middle income countries, it has just too small profit margin over the standard, monthly required-to-purchase tools.

For instance an average Type 1 Diabetic person needs:

1. Blood sugar meter tool
2. Needle for the blood sugar meter
3. Strips for the blood sugar meter
4. Daily insulin
5. Insulin for the night
6. Needles for insulin injection

From these six cost centers five of them are regular, continuous costs. For example if your blood sugar meter has a 50 pieces of test stripe pack and you have to measure your sugar at least seven times a day then it hardly lasts for one week. Not to mention the needles which you throw away after every single use for hygienic purpose.

It is a big business to offer supplies for Diabetic people and because of this there are many, flowering "*conspiracy theories*".

One of the most popular is fueled by the media, since almost every month a promising new Diabetes cure or research result is presented, although most of these researches are fading away and going into silence after the successful animal tests and clinical trials.

Many suggest that pharmaceutical companies have a joint interest to keep the Diabetes and their treatment equipment around the longest possible.

From business logic this is an understandable viewpoint. Selling a product once or re-selling it every two weeks is a huge difference in the annual income balance. Let's face the truth, there is not enough money to be made in a cure that uses an inexpensive and generically available vaccine.

And this is the point where we often forget to be human, especially if you know the story of the discovery of insulin.

So this is the main idea behind the conspiracy theory. Although does this really mean that the pharmaceutical companies never work on the cure researches in order to just focus on their potential best interests? I am not sure about this.

Hopefully there are still companies and/or private individuals who are motivated by the possible honour to eliminate an ancient disease and to find a cure which effects this many people around the World.

Truth to be told I also approached some of the major pharmaceutical companies which are providing essential supplies for people living with Diabetes. I was pretty confident that they would be open to provide information for a free education book to the fellow sufferers.

I got very prompt answers and I had to experience the bitter sweet taste of rejection. No matter how I tried to explain them that this book is free, it is educational, and more importantly I do not request any financial support, they just kept rejecting the concept saying that they are not interested to be presented in a book which is talking about "*the way towards cure*" and current Diabetes researches, not even for free. Shame.

I do not judge anyone although I learnt the lesson.

Personally, I believe *(and this is my own human nature)* that the one who will find the cure will be celebrated and immortalized, which prestige and honour is worth much more than any financial gain.

Not to mention and I put this into a silent remark, that even if the cure of the Type 1 Diabetes will be announced officially, Type 2 Diabetes will still exist since it is a lifestyle related disease.

Maybe I am a bit naive and too human. Time will tell.

The honest thing is that developing any new molecule or vaccine to the market takes millions of dollars, multi stages and at least 7-9 years from the very first test to the final market approval.

Despite the financial and regulatory considerations there are many promising ways to find the cure and some of them are already available for patients with critical conditions.

Pre-Diabetes

The underlying magic of the treatment and cure of the Pre-Diabetic state is truly rely on the willingness of the individuals.

With proper education, eating habits, physical activity, weight management and lifestyle, the risk of developing Type 2 Diabetes Mellitus is reduced.

Blood glucose levels can be managed by the healthy eating and physical activity guidelines as an individual with normal blood glucose levels, however some minor modifications may be required.

These variations depend on the individual, but it may include a decrease in the amount of carbohydrates consumed.

The consumption of alcohol should also be limited, but moderate drinking may be protective. Vegetables and fruit should be consumed in the largest proportions.

Regular physical activity has the potential to reduce insulin resistance and help decrease elevated blood glucose levels.

Worse case scenario Metformin has been proven effective in preventing the onset of diabetes.

Unfortunately Metformin is rarely being used for Diabetes prevention among people at risk for developing it. This is something that patients and doctors need to be talking about and thinking about.

Type 1

A variety of immunological approaches have been successful at preventing a disease similar to human Type 1 Diabetes in laboratory animals. As a result, hope has emerged that analogous interventions in humans might prevent Type 1 Diabetes or significantly slow the decline in beta cell function that characterizes the condition.

Just recently in 2016, scientists solve immune system mystery for Type 1 Diabetes a decades-old medical mystery by finally identifying a previously unknown molecule which is attacked by the immune system in people with Type 1 Diabetes.

The ground-breaking research, led by Dr Michael Christie from the University of Lincoln, UK, could now lead to better identification of individuals at risk of Type 1 Diabetes and inform the development of new therapies which could prevent the disease developing.

Type 1 Diabetes develops when the body is unable to produce insulin, a substance required to regulate blood sugar levels by moving glucose out of the blood and into cells to be used for energy. It is an autoimmune disease, where the body's defence system that normally protects against infections attacks and destroys the insulin-producing cells in the pancreas.

In Type 1 Diabetes, the immune system reacts to particular molecules in the pancreas, called autoantigens that it would normally ignore. People with Type 1 Diabetes have antibodies in their blood that are specific to each of the molecules.

Tests are currently used to detect these antibodies: the more antibodies detected, the higher the risk a person has of developing Type 1 Diabetes. The tests are currently used to identify those most at risk of Type 1 Diabetes, and in the future could provide an opportunity to intervene and stop the disease in its tracks.

Until now, scientists had found four molecules that are attacked by the immune system in Type 1 Diabetes. The identity of a fifth molecule – known only as "*Glima*" for the past 20 years – has been a mystery.

Dr Christie's team have successfully identified this fifth molecule as Tetraspanin-7, which could make tests for predicting Type 1 Diabetes more accurate. They are now searching for ways to block the immune attack, in order to prevent Type 1 Diabetes from developing in those at a high risk.

Being able to detect circulating autoantibodies and identify their molecular targets has allowed scientists to develop tests for the clinical diagnosis of Type 1 Diabetes, and for the identification of individuals at high risk of developing the disease.

Evidence from both animal studies and human trials indicate that Type 1 Diabetes may be prevented in individuals at risk, and a number of therapies to interfere with immune responses have proved effective in preventing disease development in animals and in slowing the loss of insulin-secreting cell function in human patients.

Screening for antibodies against the four molecules found in the pancreas is currently used to assess a person's risk of Type 1 Diabetes. Following Dr Christie's research, Tetraspanin-7 antibodies could now be included in this process. This could make tests more accurate and help researchers to understand a person's individual and unique immune response - both of which are crucial in the development of treatments that can stop the progression of Type 1 Diabetes.

Also there are various prevention trials all around the World with different approaches.

Primary prevention trials involving dietary modification have been conducted with infants identified through genetic screening as being at highest risk of developing Type 1 Diabetes.

Tested interventions and factors have included early exposure to cows' milk, the age of introduction of solid foods, supplementation with an omega-3 fatty acid, and supplementation with vitamin D. None of the trials has shown a reduction in Type 1 Incidence.

Other trials have focused on relatives of people with Type 1 Diabetes. Two large randomized clinical trials have explored the use of vitamin B6 supplementation in adults and children who are related to people with Type 1 Diabetes and are pancreatic islet antibody-positive with negative results.

Injected insulin and oral insulin have also been explored as preventive interventions in children with antibodies to insulin. The overall results were negative but a subgroup with the highest concentration of anti-insulin antibodies at the start of the trial showed some delay in onset.

Other approaches, as yet unsuccessful, have been treatment of people at high risk with nasal insulin, low-dose cyclosporine and with a monoclonal antibody.

Pancreas transplantation

In some cases, a pancreas transplant can restore proper glucose regulation therefore a pancreas transplant is occasionally considered for people with Type 1 Diabetes who have severe complications of their disease.

In most cases, pancreas transplantation is performed on individuals with Type 1 Diabetes with end-stage renal disease, Brittle Diabetes and Hypoglycaemia unawareness.

The majority of pancreas transplantation *(>90%)* are simultaneous pancreas-kidney transplantation. It may also be performed as part of a kidney-pancreas transplantation because of end stage kidney disease.

A pancreas transplant is an organ transplant that involves implanting a healthy pancreas *(one that can produce insulin)* into a person who usually has Diabetes. Because the pancreas is a vital organ, performing functions necessary in the digestion process, the recipient's native pancreas is left in place, and the donated pancreas is attached in a different location.

The surgery and accompanying immunosuppression required may be more dangerous than continued insulin replacement therapy, so is generally only used with or some time after a kidney transplant.

One reason for this is that introducing a new kidney requires taking immunosuppressive drugs such as cyclosporine. Nevertheless, this allows the introduction of a new pancreas to a person with Diabetes without any additional immunosuppressive therapy.

However, pancreas transplants alone may be beneficial in people with extremely labile Type 1 Diabetes Mellitus.

The healthy pancreas comes from a donor who has just died or it may be a partial pancreas from a living donor. At present, pancreas transplants are usually performed in persons with insulin-dependent Diabetes who can develop severe complications.

There are four main types of pancreas transplantation:

- Pancreas transplant alone, for the patient with Type 1 Diabetes who usually has severe, frequent Hypoglycemia, but adequate kidney function.
- Simultaneous pancreas-kidney transplant *(SPK)*, when the pancreas and kidney are transplanted simultaneously from the same deceased donor.
- Pancreas-after-kidney transplant *(PAK)*, when a cadaveric, or deceased, donor pancreas transplant is performed after a previous, and different, living or deceased donor kidney transplant.
- Simultaneous deceased donor pancreas and live donor kidney *(SPLK)* has the benefit of lower rate of delayed graft function than SPK and significantly reduced waiting times, resulting in improved outcomes.

Patients with the most common- and deadliest- form of pancreatic cancer *(pancreatic adenomas which are usually always malignant, with a poor prognosis and high risk for metastasis as opposed to more treatable pancreatic neuroendocrine tumors or pancreatic insulinomas)* are usually not eligible for valuable pancreatic transplantations, since the condition usually has a very high mortality rate and the disease, which is usually highly malignant and detected too late to treat, could and probably would soon return.

In the event of rejection of the new pancreas which would quickly cause life-threatening Diabetes, the recipient could not survive without the native pancreas still in place. This is also the reason for the recommended simultaneous pancreas-kidney transplantation.

The prognosis after pancreas transplantation is very good. Over the recent years, long-term success has improved and risks have decreased.

One year after transplantation more than 95% of all patients are still alive and 80-85% of all pancreases are still functional. After transplantation patients need lifelong immunosuppression.

However we should not forget that immunosuppression increases the risk for a number of different kinds of infection and cancer.

Artificial pancreas

A new device is about to change the lives of children and adults living with Type 1 diabetes. The breakthrough is so historic, patients and even doctors are getting emotional about it.

Type 1 Diabetes is a 24-hour, 7-days a week job for the diabetic and parents. Every bit of food, every activity has to be monitored and can affect blood sugar. And you can not underestimate the stress of fluctuating blood sugars and the mental stress of being your own pancreas.

Blood sugar also tends to dip dangerously low when a diabetic is asleep. Some can slip into comas or even die.

The artificial pancreas system takes the human element, and the human error, out of the equation.

A sensor and insulin pump work together to continually check a diabetic's blood sugar and automatically set it at a normal range. So every minute, it's calculating how much insulin to give.

Researchers are hoping to get the final FDA approval in 2016.

Cure through Replacing Insulin-producing Cells

Replacing Insulin-producing cells may be an option for some people with Type 1 Diabetes that are not well controlled with insulin.

It involves a 44% of success rates, defined as not needing insulin at 3 years follow the procedure occurred in.

Having Type 1 Diabetes insulin-producing beta cells are attacked by our own immune system leading to life-long dependency on daily injections of insulin. Human pluripotent stem cells *(both embryonic and induced)* not only provide tools to further our understanding of human embryonic development, but they also offer a rich source of cells to replace dead or dysfunctional cells in various traumas and degenerative diseases.

The self-renewing capacity of human pluripotent stem cells *(hPSCs)* and their ability to make most of our cell types, including insulin-producing beta cells, has inspired many laboratories *(academic and private)* to develop methods for manufacturing glucose-responsive beta cells in the laboratory.

Stem cells in the pancreas which can turn into insulin-producing cells have been identified by researchers from the Walter and Eliza Hall Institute of Medical Research, Australia.

They published their breakthrough in PLoS One *(November 9th, 2012)* and their finding raises the hope that one day soon patients with Type 1 Diabetes will be able to produce their own insulin in their own regenerated beta cells in the pancreas.

The scientists identified and isolated stem cells from the adult pancreas. They then developed a method for making them become insulin-producing cells that can secrete insulin in response to glucose in the bloodstream.

Difficulties include finding donors that are a compatible, getting the new islets to survive, and the side effects from the medications used to prevent rejection.

Currently there are many ongoing stem cell researches all around the Globe. For example Pluripotent stem cells can be used to generate beta cells but previously these cells did not function as well as normal beta cells.

In 2014 a pioneering technique was developed to transform skin cells in mice into pancreatic cells. When these cells were injected into mice with Diabetes, the animals' blood sugar levels returned to normal and they released insulin in response to blood sugar.

The power of regenerative medicine is that it can potentially provide an unlimited source of functional, insulin-producing beta cells however before these techniques can be used in humans more evidence of safety and effectiveness is needed.

Also transplanting insulin-producing islet cells into a person with Type 1 Diabetes could be a life-changing treatment for some, but transplant rejection is still a challenge.

However researchers already found one potential way to hide the transplanted islet cells from the immune system, without the need for immuno-suppressant drugs that can come with harmful side effects.

If successful, it could open exciting possibilities for people with Type 1 Diabetes.

But to demonstrate the problem there was another research whereby introducing caerulein to the pancreas of mice it was able to generate new beta cell, restore the body's ability to produce insulin. This is potentially freeing patients from daily doses of insulin to manage their blood-sugar levels.

However the problem was a slight difference between mice and humans. When caerulein is administered to humans it can cause pancreatitis.

Cure through Vaccines and Immunotherapy

There are several medications used to treat Diabetes which are working effectively by lowering blood sugar levels. Also there are a number of different classes of anti-diabetic medications. Some of these available in an oral form and others are only available by injection.

These medications can treat almost every type of the Diabetes Mellitus, except the Type 1 Diabetes which can only be treated with insulin.

As an insulin treatment Type 1 Diabetics are using typically a combination of regular and NPH insulin *(Neutral Protamine Hagedorn, an intermediate-acting insulin)*, or synthetic insulin analogs.

A few years ago there were a great hope to create a new vaccine which can treat and/or prevent Type 1 Diabetes.

The vaccine was designed to induce immune tolerance to insulin or pancreatic beta cells. The Phase II clinical trials of a vaccine containing alum and recombinant GAD65, an autoantigen involved in Type 1 Diabetes.

The research trial was highly promising until the year of 2014, when Phase III had failed.

As of 2014, other approaches such as a DNA vaccine encoding proinsulin and a peptide fragment of insulin, were in early clinical development.

Cure through Probiotic pill

Scientists claim that both Type 1 Diabetes and Type 2 Diabetes could be cured by a daily probiotic pill that "*rewires*" the body.

The new drug, which contains live bacteria from the human gut, has been shown to drastically lower blood sugar levels.

The pancreas is the organ which controls glucose levels in the body in healthy individuals, but scientists at Cornell University in New York discovered a protein secreted from a human probiotic could shift that control from the pancreas to the upper intestine.

Professor John March's team engineered a strain of lactobacillus, a human probiotic commonly found in the gut to secrete a peptide, a hormone that releases insulin in response to food entering the body.

The scientists found the cells in the upper intestine of the diabetic rats given the treatment were converted into cells that acted similarly to pancreatic cells which in healthy people secrete insulin to maintain and balance glucose levels.

The breakthrough, which relies on "*rewiring*" the body, could pave the way for a cure for both Type 1 and Type 2 Diabetes.

The promise is to just take the pill and you would not have to do anything else to control your Diabetes.

The next step would be to test higher doses of the treatment to establish if the probiotic could reverse the condition altogether.

Type 2

Type 2 Diabetes might be treatable even without serious medications. For example there are many people who managed to get rid of their symptoms through a combination of exercise, diet and body weight control.

> ***Facts & Myths*** *Nr 12.*
>
> *Myth:* Diabetics cannot eat bread, potatoes or pasta
>
> *Fact:* People with Diabetes can eat starchy foods. However, they must keep an eye on the size of the portions. Whole grain starchy foods are better, as is the case for people without Diabetes.

Facilities for Diabetes diagnosis and management should be available in primary health-care settings, with an established referral and back-referral system.

The proper care and treatment for Type 2 Diabetic people is highly important since people with Type 2 Diabetes are much more likely to develop cardiovascular diseases, such as coronary heart disease, stroke, hypertension, inflammatory heart disease and other cardiovascular conditions. Treatments tend to be similar to the ones used on patients who do not have Diabetes.

Implementing the concept of "Balanced life"

Management and the possibility to be cured from Type 2 Diabetes includes:

1. Healthy eating
2. Regular exercise
3. Possibly, Diabetes medication or insulin therapy
4. Blood sugar monitoring

These steps will help keep your blood sugar level closer to normal, which can delay or prevent complications.

Healthy eating

Healthy eating does not mean to eat less, but to eat well. And this starts already in the young age. Studies shows that teens who skip breakfast increase their risk of obesity and diabetes later in life. 68% of the freshly diagnosed Type 2 Diabetic people ate little or nothing in their childhood for breakfast.

Despite the popular belief there is no specific diet for Type 2 Diabetic people.

What is really important is to create and centre your diet around high-fibre and low-fat foods, such as fruits, vegetables and whole grains.

You have to reduce the eating of refined carbohydrates, sweets and try to eat fewer animal products.

It is recommended to look for the low glycemic index foods. The glycemic index is a measure of how quickly a food causes a rise in your blood sugar. Foods with a high glycemic index raise your blood sugar quickly. Low glycemic index foods may help you achieve a more stable blood sugar. Foods with a low glycemic index typically are foods that are higher in fiber.

***Facts & Myths** Nr 13.*

Myth: Diabetes diets are different from other people's

Fact: The diet doctors and specialized nutritionists recommend for Diabetes patients are healthy ones; healthy for everybody, including people without the disease.

Meals should contain plenty of vegetables, fruit, whole grains, and they should be low in salt and sugar, and saturated or trans fat.

Experts say that there is no need to buy special diabetic foods because they offer no special benefit, compared to the healthy things we can buy in most shops.

If you are not confident about your meal plane, a registered dietitian can help you put together a meal plan that fits your health goals, food preferences and lifestyle. He or she can also teach you how to monitor your carbohydrate intake and let you know about how many carbohydrates you need to eat with your meals and snacks to keep your blood sugar levels more stable.

Some studies also suggest that various foods has beta cell regenerative potential that can be the favor of Diabetes symptom management. These foods are capable of stimulating beta cell regeneration within the pancreas, and as a result may be potentially provide a cure for Type 2 Diabetes.

Natural substances that are experimentally confirmed to stimulate beta cell regeneration: Arginine, Avocado, Berberine, Chard, Corn Silk, Curcumin, Genistein, Honey, Nigella Sativa, Stevia.

Cinnamon might be also helpful in the blood sugar control.

However healthy eating does not always means what you think first. In 2014 a finding was publish stating that the compounds found in herbs, berries, red grapes, and red wine may protects against Diabetes. That is because they are linked to lower insulin resistance and better control of blood sugar.

This exciting finding shows that some components of foods that we consider unhealthy like chocolate or wine may contain some beneficial substances. Yes, it is also believed that chocolate could help to reduce the risk of heart disease.

Not to mention that increasing your daily consumption of coffee may help protect against diabetes. Researched proved that individuals who increased their daily coffee intake by more than one cup over a four-year period had an 11 percent lower risk of developing Type 2 Diabetes.

Although in a second round the researchers found that changing coffee consumption either increasing the risk for Diabetes or lowering it. It depends on the individuals. So coffee is not a miracle "*drug*" by any means, and it is important not to drink too much of it, although in some cases it might help you.

Talking about drinks another study suggests replacing soft drinks and sweetened milky drinks with water or unsweetened tea or coffee is practical way to reduce rising incidence of disease by up to a quarter.

Basically you have the potential to reduce the burden of diabetes by reducing the percentage of energy consumed from sweet beverages.

Regular exercise

Any human being needs regular exercise in their lives. It is recommended to have at least of 150 minutes of combined physical exercise in a week. This can be walk, work, aerobic, etc. because physical activity lowers blood sugar.

For Type 2 Diabetics the minimum recommended fitness or aerobic activity is 30 minutes a day, such as walking, swimming and biking. Choose activities you enjoy and if you have not been active for a while, start slowly and build up gradually.

Combined exercises *(such as dance)* often gives you much joy and helps control blood sugar more effectively than either type of exercise alone. And there are various possibilities both for women and men.

Some examples of aerobic activities:

- Brisk walking *(outside or inside on a treadmill)*
- Bicycling/Stationary cycling indoors
- Dancing
- Low-impact aerobics
- Swimming or water aerobics
- Playing tennis
- Stair climbing
- Jogging/Running
- Hiking
- Rowing
- Ice-skating or roller-skating
- Cross-country skiing
- Moderate-to-heavy gardening

Also some ideas for strength training activities:

- Weight machines or free weights at the gym
- Using resistance bands
- Lifting light weights or objects like canned goods or water bottles at home
- Calisthenics or exercises that use your own body weight to work your muscles *(examples are pushups, sit ups, squats, lunges, wall-sits and planks)*
- Classes that involve strength training
- Other activities that build and keep muscle like heavy gardening

It is important to check your blood sugar level before any activity. You might need to eat a snack before exercising to help prevent low blood sugar if you take Diabetes medications that lower your blood sugar.

Also it can be a good idea to discuss your chosen activity with your doctor or Diabetes specialist.

Monitoring your blood sugar

It goes without any word that it is the most important task you have. Depending on your treatment plan, you may need to check and record your blood sugar level every now and then or, if you are on insulin, multiple times a day.

Careful monitoring is the only way to make sure that your blood sugar level remains within your target range.

Sometimes, blood sugar levels can be unpredictable. With help from your Diabetes treatment team, you will learn how your blood sugar level changes in response to food, exercise, alcohol, illness and medication.

Reversing Type 2 Diabetes in Barbados

Barbados has a 19% prevalence of Diabetes among adults. One in three adults is obese; two out of three are overweight or obese; and under one in 10 adults eats five or more portions of fresh fruit and vegetables a day.

The Barbados Diabetes Reversal Study is designed to test the feasibility of an 8-week, low-calorie diet, with follow-up support for 6 months on diet and physical activity, to reverse Type 2 Diabetes.

Ten men and 15 women aged 26–68 years participated in the study.

All had been diagnosed with Type 2 Diabetes in the previous 6 years, none was on insulin, and their body mass indices ranged from 27–53. All glucose-lowering medication ceased at the start of the study.

Participants consumed a predominantly liquid diet consisting of four portions a day, each of 190 calories. Participants were also encouraged to eat low-carbohydrate, high-fibre vegetables.

By week 8, average weight loss was 10 kg. Several people saw improvements in blood glucose levels and in blood pressure. Three months after finishing the 8-week diet, 17 participants had Fasting Plasma Glucose *(FPG)* below the diagnostic threshold for Diabetes compared to three at the start, and despite remaining off glucose-lowering medication. For nine of the 12 participants on medication for hypertension at the start of the study, blood pressure fell sufficiently that they could stop taking hypertension medication by the 8th week.

Participants have so far articulated several challenges in participating in the study, including the monotony of the low-calorie diet phase, the high cost of fresh fruits and vegetables, and feeling poorly equipped to prepare non-starchy vegetables, even with provided recipes. There was resounding agreement that the most challenging times are in social settings, where there is peer pressure to consume food and drink.

A key element of the programme's success has been the support participants have received from family, friends and each other *(particularly through the use of social media)*. However, their experiences also demonstrate the everyday difficulties of undertaking this approach in a context of widespread obesity.

Basic medications for Type 2 Diabetes

If you have Type 2 Diabetes, then it is highly possible to achieve your target blood sugar levels with a lifestyle change including proper diet and exercise only. Although many Type 2 Diabetes patients may also need Diabetes medications or in worse case insulin therapy.

The decision about which medications are best depends on many factors, including your blood sugar level and any other health problems you have. Your doctor might even combine drugs from different classes to help you control your blood sugar in several different ways.

There are several classes of anti-diabetic medications available.

➡ **Metformin** *(Glucophage, Glumetza)* is generally recommended as a first line treatment and prescribed drug for Type 2 Diabetes as there is some evidence that it decreases mortality, however this conclusion is questioned.

It works by improving the sensitivity of your body tissues to insulin so that your body uses insulin more effectively.

Your doctor will also recommend lifestyle changes, such as losing weight and becoming more active.

Nausea and diarrhea are possible side effects of Metformin. These side effects usually go away as your body gets used to the medicine.

Metformin also lowers glucose production in the liver and it should not be used in those with severe kidney or liver problems.

If Metformin and lifestyles changes are not sufficient enough to control your blood sugar level, other oral or injected medications can be added after three months.

Other classes of medications might include:

➡ **Sulfonylureas**: These medications help your body secrete more insulin. Possible side effects include low blood sugar and weight gain.

Examples of medications in this class include Glyburide *(DiaBeta, Glynase)*, Glipizide *(Glucotrol)* and Glimepiride *(Amaryl)*.

- **Meglitinides**: These medications work like Sulfonylureas by stimulating the pancreas to secrete more insulin, but they're faster acting, and the duration of their effect in the body is shorter. They also have a risk of causing low blood sugar, but this risk is lower than with sulfonylureas.

  Weight gain is a possibility with this class of medications as well. Examples include Repaglinide *(Prandin)* and Nateglinide *(Starlix)*.

- **Thiazolidinediones**: Like Metformin, these medications make the body's tissues more sensitive to insulin.

  This class of medications has been linked to weight gain and other more-serious side effects, such as an increased risk of heart failure and fractures.
  Because of these risks, these medications generally are not a first-choice treatment.

  Rosiglitazone *(Avandia)* and Pioglitazone *(Actos)* are examples of Thiazolidinediones.

  However it is important to know that Rosiglitazone, has not been found to improve long-term outcomes even though it improves blood sugar levels. Additionally it is associated with increased rates of heart disease and death.

- **Dipeptidyl Peptidase-4 Inhibitors** *(DPP-4)*: These medications help reduce blood sugar levels, but tend to have a modest effect. They do not cause weight gain.

  Examples of these medications are Sitagliptin *(Januvia)*, Saxagliptin *(Onglyza)* and Linagliptin *(Tradjenta)*.

- **Glucagon-Like Peptide-1 receptor agonists** *(GLP-1)*: These medications slow digestion and help lower blood sugar levels, though not as much as Sulfonylureas. Their use is often associated with some weight loss.

This class of medications is not recommended for use by itself.

Exenatide *(Byetta)* and Liraglutide *(Victoza)* are examples of GLP-1 receptor agonists. Possible side effects include nausea and an increased risk of pancreatitis.

Liraglutide *(or Victoza)* is a relatively new GLP-1 analogue used to treat Type 2 Diabetes. Liraglutide functions in two ways: it stimulates insulin production and suppresses glucagon production.

Liraglutide, which is injected once a day, lowers blood glucose levels both after meals and while fasting, making it easier for people with Type 2 Diabetes to manage their Diabetes. Liraglutide also improves weight loss and more interestingly it helps with memory loss as well as a possible new treat drug for Alzheimer's.

- **SGLT2 inhibitors**: These are the newest Diabetes drugs on the market. They work by preventing the kidneys from reabsorbing sugar into the blood. Instead, the sugar is excreted in the urine.

  Examples include Canagliflozin *(Invokana)* and Dapagliflozin *(Farxiga)*. Side effects may include yeast infections and urinary tract infections, increased urination and hypotension.

- **Insulin therapy**: Injections of insulin may either be added to oral medication or used alone. Most people do not initially need insulin.

In the past, insulin therapy was used as a very last resort for the treatment of Type 2 Diabetes, but today it is often prescribed sooner because of its benefits.

Because normal digestion interferes with insulin taken by mouth, insulin recommended to be injected, although there are inhalable insulin as well available for those who are afraid of needles or whom prefers to take the insulin in a much sophisticated way in public areas.

Depending on your needs, your doctor may prescribe a mixture of insulin types. When insulin therapy is used, a long-acting formulation is typically added at night, with oral medications being continued.

Doses are then increased to effect *(blood sugar levels being well controlled)*. When nightly insulin is insufficient, twice daily insulin may achieve better control.

The long acting insulins Glargine and Detemir are equally safe and effective, and do not appear much better than neutral protamine Hagedorn *(NPH)* insulin, but as they are significantly more expensive, they are not cost effective as of 2010.

Insulin injections involve using a fine needle and syringe or an insulin pen injector, a device that looks similar to an ink pen except the cartridge is filled with insulin.

There are many types of insulin, and they each work in a different way.

- ➡ Insulin glulisine *(Apidra)*
- ➡ Insulin lispro *(Humalog)*
- ➡ Insulin aspart *(Novolog)*
- ➡ Insulin glargine *(Lantus)*
- ➡ Insulin detemir *(Levemir)*
- ➡ Insulin isophane *(Humulin N, Novolin N)*

Always better to discuss the pros and cons of different drugs with your Diabetes doctor. Together you can decide which medication is best for you after considering many factors, including costs and other aspects of your health.

In addition to Diabetes medications your doctor might prescribe low-dose aspirin therapy as well as blood pressure and cholesterol-lowering medications to help prevent heart and blood vessel disease.

Also for those woman are **pregnant** and they have Type 2 Diabetes insulin is generally the treatment of choice during pregnancy.

Cholesterol-lowering medications and some blood pressure drugs can not be used during pregnancy and many women with Type 2 Diabetes will require insulin therapy during pregnancy. Visit your ophthalmologist during the first trimester of your pregnancy and at one year postpartum.

Alternative medicines

It is not a cure suggestion, more like a warning that no alternative treatments can cure Diabetes.

Even if numerous alternative medicine substances have been shown to improve insulin sensitivity in some studies, other studies fail to find any benefit for blood sugar control or in lowering A1C levels.

Because of the conflicting findings, no alternative therapies are recommended to help with blood sugar management.

It is critical that people who are using insulin therapy for Diabetes do not stop using insulin unless directed to do so by their physicians.

If you decide to try an alternative therapy do not stop taking the medications that your doctor has prescribed.

Be sure to discuss the use of any of these alternative medicines therapies with your doctor to make sure that they will not cause adverse reactions or interact with your current medications.

Marijuana

Medical marijuana is among the most researched next-generation medicines.

For example GW Pharmaceuticals studying the ways to use the chemical compounds found in marijuana since 1998.

So does this means that we all should circulate the marijuana cigarettes and enjoy some weed? Not necessarily.

What GW Pharmaceuticals thinks is that medical marijuana may have a chance for greater success, offering a new way in Diabetes treatment.

They has already conducted a pre-clinical trial and an early stage trial of its cannabis-based drug GWP42004.

In the pre-clinical animal studies, followed by a small human trial that showed that GWP42004 may help Type 2 Diabetics improve fasting glucose levels, lower blood pressure, and improve pancreatic cell function.

A phase 2 trial started in 2014-2015.

Protein injection

FGF1 could revolutionize Diabetes treatment.

Controlling glucose is a dominant problem in our society and when mice with the human equivalent of Type 2 Diabetes were injected with the protein FGF1, their blood sugar levels returned to normal over two days.

Just one injection of the protein both regulated these levels and even helped reverse insulin insensitivity, the underlying cause of Diabetes.

As the result of the research Ronald M. Evans, director of Salk's Gene Expression Laboratory said that FGF1 offers a new method to control glucose in a powerful and unexpected way.

Hoping to find better options for Diabetes patients, Evans and his team decided to study FGF1 after they discovered that the protein can help the body respond to insulin. They became interested in therapeutic uses of the protein when they noticed that mice lacking the FGF1 gene became diabetic when placed on a high-fat diet.

In addition to being effective against diabetes, the protein has several advantages over current Diabetes drugs. It does not result in dangerous side effects seen with other Diabetes drugs, such as heart problems, weight gain, or Hypoglycemia.

Additionally, FGF1 not only increased insulin levels but also helped the mice regain their own ability to regulate insulin.

Surgical ways for Type 2 patients

Gastric bypass surgery can reverse Type 2 Diabetes in a high proportion of patients.

It is important to note that a Bariatric surgery can be only successful if the patient is committed to change on his/her lifestyle. It is a sad statistic that within three to five years the Type 2 Diabetes disease recurs in approximately 21% of them because of the lack of willingness for a healthy and balanced life.

The good news is that the blood sugar levels return to normal in 55% to 95% of people with Type 2 Diabetes, depending on the procedure performed. This percentage is influenced by a longstanding history of Type 2 Diabetes before the surgery.

If you are convinced in this way and you consulted with your doctors, the two basic requirements for the surgery are:

➡ Having Type 2 Diabetes

➡ The Body Mass Index *(BMI)* should be greater than 35

It is recommended that this option be considered in those who are unable to get both their weight and blood sugar under control.

Drawbacks to the surgery include its high cost, and there are risks involved, including a risk of death.

For the success, drastic lifestyle changes are required and long-term complications may include nutritional deficiencies and osteoporosis.

Type 3

In the past years researchers also discovered that some of the **Diabetes medication** actually **could treat Alzheimer's**.

Researchers are also testing various Diabetes medication as potential treatments for the neurodegenerative disease.

Incretin mimetic drugs, such as Liraglutide *(Victoza)* and Lixisenatide *(Lyxumia)* have shown potential for preventing the development of Alzheimer's disease are being investigated as a possible treatment.

Researchers discovered that the Diabetes drug Liraglutide reduced the damage caused by dementia in mice. Now Liraglutide's restorative effects are being trialled on over 200 men and women in their 50s.

Pioglitazone *(Actos)* has shown evidence that it may also help towards preventing the development of Alzheimer's disease.

An experimental Diabetes drug known as (Val8)GLP-1 could help combat the effects of Alzheimer's disease, according to scientists who say the drug may be able to protect damaged brain cells and promote the growth of new ones.

The University of Ulster researchers tested the drug on healthy mice and examined its effects on the brain. (Val8)GLP-1 works by simulating the activity of the GLP-1 protein in the brain to help the body control its response to blood sugar.

The team found it entered the brain and promoted new cell growth in the hippocampus, which is the area involved in short and long-term memory.

In addition, they reported that blocking the effect of GLP-1 in the brains of the mice led to poorer performance in learning and memory tasks, while boosting it with the drug appeared to have no effect on behavior. It also had no side-effects at the doses tested, they added.

The findings suggest that as well as its role in insulin signaling, GLP-1 may also be important for the production of new nerve cells in the brain.

Also researchers from Imperial College London recently recruited people with early Alzheimers disease for a trial of a Diabetes drug.

If successful, **the drug could reverse the damage caused by Alzheimer's disease**.

The study, which will cost £5million, could lead to the biggest breakthrough in the treatment of dementia for over decades.

Prevention of Diabetes

"KNOWLEDGE GAINED FROM PROOF-OF-CONCEPT STUDIES, OR BOOKS SUCH AS THIS ONE AS WELL CONFIRMS THAT TYPE 2 DIABETES CAN BE DELAYED OR PREVENTED, BUT TURNING THIS KNOWLEDGE INTO LARGE-SCALE IMPACT BRINGS SIGNIFICANT CHALLENGES."

Type 1 Diabetes cannot be prevented with current knowledge. Effective approaches are available to prevent Type 2 Diabetes, it can often be prevented by a person being a normal body weight, physical exercise, and following a healthful diet. This can also prevent the complications and premature death that can result from all types of Diabetes.

These include policies and practices across whole populations and within specific settings *(school, home, workplace)* that contribute to good health for everyone, regardless of whether they have Diabetes, such as exercising regularly, eating healthily, avoiding smoking and controlling blood pressure and lipids.

Taking a life-course perspective is essential for preventing Type 2 Diabetes, as it is for many health conditions. Early in life when eating and physical activity habits are formed and when the long-term regulation of energy balance may be programmed, there is a critical window for intervention to mitigate the risk of obesity and Type 2 Diabetes later in life.

Dietary changes known to be effective in helping to prevent Diabetes include a diet rich in whole grains and fiber, and choosing good fats, such as polyunsaturated fats found in nuts, vegetable oils, and fish. Limiting sugary beverages and eating less red meat and other sources of saturated fat can also help in the prevention of Diabetes.

Active smoking is also associated with an increased risk of Diabetes, so smoking cessation can be an important preventive measure as well.

The World Health Organization estimates that, globally, 422 million adults aged over 18 years were living with Diabetes in 2014.

The number of people with Diabetes *(defined in surveys as those having a fasting plasma glucose value of greater than or equal to 7.0 mmol/L or on medication for Diabetes/raised blood glucose)* has steadily risen over the past few decades, due to population growth, the increase in the average age of the population, and the rise in prevalence of Diabetes at each age. Worldwide, the number of people with Diabetes has substantially increased between 1980 and 2014, rising from 108 million to current numbers that are around four times higher.

No single policy or intervention can ensure this happens. It calls for a whole-of-government and whole-of-society approach, in which all sectors systematically consider the health impact of policies in trade, agriculture, nance, transport, education and urban planning, recognizing that health is enhanced or obstructed as a result of policies in these and other areas.

For older adults the same amount of physical activity is recommended, but should also include balance and muscle strengthening activity tailored to their ability and circumstances.

Recommended physical activities by the World Health Organization:

- ➡ It is recommended that children and youth aged 5–17 years should do at least 60 minutes of moderate- to vigorous-intensity physical activity daily.
- ➡ It is recommended that adults aged 18–64 years should do at least 150 minutes of moderate-intensity aerobic physical

activity *(for example brisk walking, jogging, gardening)* spread throughout the week, or at least 75 minutes of vigorous-intensity aerobic physical activity throughout the week, or an equivalent combination of moderate- and vigorous-intensity activity.

Consumer awareness and knowledge of healthy diet and physical activity can be achieved through sustained media and educational campaigns aimed at increasing consumption of healthy foods *(or reducing consumption of less healthy ones)*, and increasing physical activity. For example, a social marketing campaign in Tonga using netball to promote physical activity among women as part of a national NCD campaign has resulted in increased participation both in netball and leisure-time physical activity by women. These campaigns have greater impact and are more cost-effective when used within multicomponent strategies

Knowledge gained from proof-of-concept studies, or books such as this one as well confirms that Type 2 Diabetes can be delayed or prevented, but turning this knowledge into large-scale impact brings significant challenges.

Global burden

"THE AVAILABILITY OF ESSENTIAL MEDICINES AND BASIC TECHNOLOGIES IS A CRITICAL COMPONENT OF DIABETES MANAGEMENT."

Even if the majority, 71% of countries have national Diabetes policies, national policies to address unhealthy diet and physical inactivity and national guidelines or standards for Diabetes management, globally an estimated 422 million adults were living with Diabetes in 2014, compared to 108 million in 1980.

The global prevalence *(age-standardized)* of Diabetes has nearly **doubled** since 1980, rising from 4.7% to **8.5% in the adult population**. Over the past decade, Diabetes prevalence has risen faster in low- and middle-income countries than in high-income countries.

Diabetes caused 1.5 million deaths in 2012. Higher-than-optimal blood glucose caused an additional 2.2 million deaths, by increasing the risks of cardiovascular and other diseases.

The majority of people with Diabetes are affected by **Type 2 Diabetes**. This used to occur nearly entirely among adults, but now occurs **in children too**.

Diabetes and its complications **bring** about **substantial economic loss to people** with Diabetes and their families, and to health systems and national economies through direct medical costs and loss of work and wages. While the major cost drivers are hospital and outpatient care, a contributing factor is the rise in cost for analogue insulins, which are increasingly prescribed despite little evidence that they provide significant advantages over cheaper human insulins.

In general, primary health-care practitioners in low-income countries do not have access to the basic technologies needed to help people with Diabetes properly manage their disease. Which could be also considered against the will of Sir Frederick Banting, the founder of insulin, who made the patent available without charge and did not attempt to control commercial production.

Not treating well people with Diabetes also limiting them to contribute to the society in their full capability.

One study estimates that losses in Gross Domestic Product *(GDP)* worldwide from 2011 to 2030, including both the direct and indirect costs of Diabetes, will total US$ 1.7 trillion, comprising US $ 900 billion for high-income countries and US$ 800 billion for low- and middle-income countries.

Therefore we can clearly state that Diabetes imposes a large economic burden on the global health-care system and the wider global economy. This burden can be measured through direct medical costs, indirect costs associated with productivity loss, premature mortality and the negative impact of Diabetes on nations' Gross Domestic Product *(GDP)*.

Based on cost estimates from a recent systematic review, it has been estimated that the direct annual cost of Diabetes to the world is more than US$ 827 billion.

The International Diabetes Federation *(IDF)* estimates that total global health-care spending on Diabetes more than tripled over the period 2003 to 2013 – the result of increases in the number of people with Diabetes and increases in per capita Diabetes spending.

Direct medical costs associated with Diabetes include expenditures for preventing and treating Diabetes and its complications. These include outpatient and emergency care, inpatient hospital care, medications and medical supplies such as injection devices and self-monitoring consumables, and long-term care.

Besides the economic burden on the health-care system and national economy, Diabetes can impose a large economic burden on people with Diabetes and their families in terms of higher out-of-pocket health-care payments and loss of family income associated with disability and premature loss of life.

Sugar-Sweetened-Beverage Tax in Mexico

The prevalence of overweight and obesity in Mexico stands at more than 33% in children and around 70% in adults. Mexico has the highest prevalence of Diabetes among Organization for Economic Cooperation and Development *(OECD)* member countries, and the highest per capita consumption of soft drinks worldwide.

In January 2014 Mexico implemented a nationwide tax on drinks containing added sugar *(bebidas azucaradas)* that increased their price by over 10%. While it is too early to draw far-reaching conclusions, one analysis estimated that the 10% increase in the price of added-sugar drinks was associated with an 11.6% decrease in the quantity consumed.

During the first year of the tax, purchases of taxed sugar-sweetened beverages decreased by an average of 6% compared to what would have been expected without implementation of the tax, with higher reductions found in households of low socioeconomic status.

The availability of essential medicines and basic technologies for early detection, diagnosis and monitoring of Diabetes in primary health-care facilities is a critical component of Diabetes management capacity.

Diabetes is recognized as an important cause of premature death and disability. It is one of four priority noncommunicable diseases *(NCDs)* targeted by world leaders in the 2011 Political Declaration on the Prevention and Control of NCDs.

The declaration recognizes that the incidence and impacts of Diabetes and other NCDs can be largely prevented or reduced with an approach that incorporates evidence-based, affordable, cost-effective, population-wide and multisectoral interventions.

To catalyze national action, the World Health Assembly adopted a comprehensive global monitoring framework in 2013, comprised of nine voluntary global targets to reach by 2025.

Countries can take a series of actions, in line with the objectives of the World Health Organization NCD Global Action Plan 2013–2020, to reduce the impact of Diabetes:

➡ Establish national mechanisms such as high-level multisectoral commissions to ensure political commitment, resource allocation, effective leadership and advocacy for an integrated NCD response, with specific attention to Diabetes.

➡ Build the capacity of ministries of health to exercise a strategic leadership role, engaging stakeholders across sectors and society. Set national targets and indicators to foster accountability. Ensure that national policies and plans addressing Diabetes are fully costed and then funded and implemented.

➡ Prioritize actions to prevent people becoming overweight and obese, beginning before birth and in early childhood. Implement policies and programmes to promote breastfeeding and the consumption of healthy foods and to discourage the consumption of unhealthy foods, such as sugary sodas. Create supportive built and social environments for physical activity. A combination of social policies, legislation, changes to the environment and raising awareness of health risks works best for promoting healthier diets and physical activity at the necessary scale.

➡ Strengthen the health system response to NCDs, including Diabetes, particularly at primary-care level. Implement guidelines and protocols to improve diagnosis and management of Diabetes in primary health care. Establish policies and programmes to ensure equitable access to essential technologies for diagnosis and management. Make essential medicines such as human insulin available and affordable to all who need them.

- ➡ Address key gaps in the Diabetes knowledge base. Outcome evaluations of innovative programmes intended to change behaviour are a particular need.
- ➡ Strengthen national capacity to collect, analyse and use representative data on the burden and trends of Diabetes and its key risk factors. Develop, maintain and strengthen a Diabetes registry if feasible and sustainable.

Everyone can play a role in reducing the impact of all forms of Diabetes. Governments, health-care providers, people with Diabetes, civil society, food producers and manufacturers and suppliers of medicines and technology are all stakeholders.

Management Sciences for Health *(MSH)* is a non-profit organization established in 1971. Since its establishment it has worked in over 150 countries to develop health systems, focusing on improving quality, availability and affordability of health services.

One of the tools developed by MSH is the International Drug Price Indicator Guide *(IDPIG)*. The guide provides a variety of prices from different sources including pharmaceutical suppliers, international development agencies and governments.

This guide allows for comparison of prices of medicines of assured quality and is used as a reference in many approaches looking at access to medicines, for example the methodology developed by World Health Organization and Health Action International.

Using the online version of IDPIG, data from 1996 to 2014 were extracted from purchasers of insulin. All insulin formulations were standardized to an equivalent of a 10 ml 100 IU vial. The minimum, maximum and median prices are calculated over the time period for all countries combined, as well as median prices over the time period, disaggregated by country income group as defined by the World Bank in 2015.

There are no simple solutions for addressing Diabetes but coordinated, multicomponent intervention can make a significant difference.

Facts & Myths *Nr 14.*

Myth: Diabetes patients are more susceptible to colds and illnesses in general

Fact: A person with Diabetes with good Diabetes control is no more likely to become ill with a cold or something else than other people.

However, when a Diabetic catches a cold, their Diabetes becomes harder to control, so they have a higher risk of complications.

Conclusions

> "EVEN IF IT WOULD NOT BE ENOUGH THAT A CHILD SUFFERS FROM A LIFE THREATENING DISEASE, MANY KINDERGARTENS REFUSE TO TAKE THESE CHILDREN, AVOIDING THE RESPONSIBILITY AND CARE TOWARDS A DIABETIC CHILD."

All types of Diabetes Mellitus are treatable. Although the numbers of people with Diabetes continue to rise because of the way we eat, move, live.

These impacts can be reduced through effective actions with global efforts. Commitments towards Sustainable Development Goals and focused attention on Diabetes prevention and management should be among the number one priorities.

A proper Diabetes prevention plan should also include proper Diabetes education from the earliest period possible.

Sadly many people have no idea about the possible risks and linked complications to the Diabetes. There is a misconception that Diabetes equals with obesity and that's all.

They often treat symptoms such as stroke or nerve damages as standalone symptoms, without taking into consideration the underlying reason, their Diabetes.

Also due to a lack of competency, information and supporting tools, many kindergartens refuse to take children with Diabetes avoiding the responsibility and care towards a Diabetic child.

It is our overall responsibility to care for 422 million people with Diabetes and take the management of this condition to a global success by allowing access to essential medicines, technologies and knowledge as well.

To ensure equitable access to affordable medicines such as the life-saving insulin or to medical devices such as a blood sugar level sensor is essential.

A human life should not be measured and dependent based on corporate profits on life saving medications.

This is also a reason why independent funds should be allocated to private companies as well, which are aiming to develop technological solutions which can offer more balanced life for people with Diabetes, without forcing them into the situation whereby they have to accept funds from the pharmaceutical companies, that might influence the outcome of the project.

There are no simple solutions for addressing Diabetes but coordinated, multicomponent intervention can make a significant difference.

Together, 422 million Diabetics and their loved ones can make a change. Just sitting in our chair waiting that someone makes our life better is not working. We can decide to die as individuals or to heal together as a big Diabetics family.

Everyone has a role to play, governments, health-care providers, people with Diabetes and those who care for them, civil societies, food producers, manufacturers and suppliers of medicines, technology companies are all stakeholders.

Collectively, we can all make a significant contribution to halt the rise in Diabetes and improve the lives of those living with this disease.

Bonus chapter:
My Type 1 Diabetes story...

"DIABETES WAS MY UNEXPECTED NEW BRIDE AND WE MADE OUR MARRIAGE IN HELL..."

Since I was diagnosed with Type 1 Diabetes I had a very personal motivation to create for you and millions of others this book and collection of knowledge on Diabetes.

Truth to be told, I am not a doctor or a healthcare professional however I believe that being a victim of Diabetes much more qualifies me than being "just" a doctor. Also I learnt during these years that money is not the prime asset in life, however health and being with your loved ones is. And believe me that Type 1 Diabetes can test you big time.

I clearly remember that I was 29 years old when I noticed that I am getting more and more thirsty. A few weeks later I started to loose some weight, more precisely it led me loosing over 20kg by the end of the second month.

Since I was 108 kg before, many friends started to give me compliments that I am in a good shape and it felt really good. I also started to feel more and more confident myself in my body, however I felt those terrible cramps in my leg during the nights. Soon the devastating pain in my leg was complimented with a very extent thirst. I started to drink 6-8 bottles of mineral water in a day which did not seem normal.

Before a very short time that I would have ended up in Diabetes coma, I was rushed to the hospital where I got the shocking news that I have Type 1 Diabetes and there is no cure to it.

I asked the doctor how is it possible that I received this life-long illness. She told me that the reason for developing Type 1 Diabetes is not known. Since I had no one in my family with Diabetes she said it was probably developed because of an increased stress or trauma.

She was probably right, because I clearly remember that I went through a difficult time back then, when one of my old business associate created a fake Facebook profile with my name. He blackmailed me first, requesting money to remove it and when I ignored him, he tried to ask money in my name from my friends and relatives. I reported him 16 times at the police, but since there was no withholding decision against him, he just continued.

This caused me a lot of stress and reputation damage which probably turned into a point where my body triggered my Diabetes.

At this point it did not matter anymore how healthy I lived before I had to realized that my life is completely changing. And it was not a positive transformation.

After spending a week in the hospital, learning all the important things about how to manage my condition, my doctor told me that I will have a "*Honeymoon*".

I looked at her as a silly donkey, because in that period I had no girlfriend in my life and her prediction seemed to be weird.

As honeymoon she referred to a 3-6 months period where the pancreas is still working but with a very low capacity. However as with any marriage I felt that this is the trap because after the honeymoon the newly wed wife takes everything over and I can loose my control over what I have.

Diabetes was my unexpected new bride and we made our marriage in Hell...

So as it was predicted after 3 months my "*new wife*" did not allow my old lifestyle. She took everything over and overwrote all my rules as she wanted.

As with 12% of Type 1 Diabetics I also went into temporary depression because of these unforeseen changes in my life.

Luckily, my ex-wife decided to help me through this period. She came down to Monaco and France where I lived and she moved in for 9 months helping me to overcome all these obstacles.

With her help I learnt again to fight for myself and for my aims instead of sinking in self pity. She made me remember how important life and my disease is effecting not just me, but all who care about me. All who are worth fighting for.

She also told me that thanks to my business experience, spending 16 years as one of the top IT business solution developer for the biggest multinational companies, including many pharmaceutical ones, I have the chance to help people with a solution.

From that moment on I started to research the disease and I started to follow many medical researches and case studies. I was ready to change the medical industry. However I had to realize that despite all the promising researches, progresses there is no cure in the pipeline yet.

This was the moment when I decided to start to create a medical solution *(http://www.diabetes-cure.me)* which offers and creates a better living quality for those who are suffering from Diabetes.

For me it is key to live a quality, healthy life and I think it summarizes all the elements I would like to reach through a solution for fellow Diabetics. And to accomplish this you do not necessary need the cure as the first step, but at least some medical tools which makes your life easier and your treatment more reliable.

Since I was really fed up with pricking my fingers seven times a day for blood samples, my very first aim was to find or develop a non-invasive, 100% pain-free Diabetes management device combined with the technological advantage of an analytics and alerting software.

During the process I met many people with so called "causes", collecting various funds in the name of Diabetes, however actually they just used the proceeds to finance their own lifestyles without a single effort to make a difference.

It is very painful to watch this for someone who actually suffers from this life-threatening condition.

For me Diabetes is not a hobby or a business which you can close. It is a life long disease, therefore to find a balanced life and to offer the same to others is my ultimate aim. Something which is driven by passion and commitment. I hope more and more people will realize at the end of the day that there is always a way to improve our life.

Focusing on the real needs of Diabetic people I truly believe that there is a chance to change the healthcare industry.

I truly hope that this book with a brief collection of some possible ways toward the cure of Diabetes triggers your desire as well to make a permanent change and maybe join us who do not sit tight and give up the hope.

And finally I would like to share with you one of my favorite story related Mother Teresa. We have lost a great humanitarian in her, but she left many things behind and one of them was a lesson for us here, now.

When Mother Teresa was awarded the Nobel Peace Prize in 1979, she said that

> *"When we work hard all day long, it feels like we are only a drop in the ocean. But if our individual drops were not in the ocean... the ocean would be dry."*

Each one of you is a drop in OUR Diabetic ocean and without each of us commonly we would be empty and dry. So please, never forget how important you are.

Thank you for reading and sharing this book.

Acknowledgements

I would like to say thank you for all the people, companies and institutions who made Diabetes knowledge available publicly.

Many of these knowledges guided me through during the writing process of present book.

I have to say a very-very special thank you to

★ World Health Organization (WHO)

★ WikiPedia

because of the extremely useful information they provided to people living with Diabetes.

During the writing of the "Diabetes: the way towards CURE" book I also learnt and developed knowledge from the following sources, thank you for that:

★ American Diabetes Association
(http://www.diabetes.org/food-and-fitness/fitness/types-of-activity/what-we-recommend.html)

★ CostCo
(http://cdiabetes.com/testing/)

★ Daily Mail & Dr Martin Scurr
(http://www.dailymail.co.uk/health/article-2715957/ASK-THE-DOCTOR-Could-stress-given-diabetes.html)

★ Daily Mail & Lizzie Parry
(http://www.dailymail.co.uk/health/article-2937602/Both-types-diabetes-CURED-daily-probiotic-pill-rewires-body-scientists-claim.html)

★ Diabetes.co.uk

★ Diabetes Daily
(https://www.diabetesdaily.com/blog/pros-and-cons-of-a-continuous-glucose-monitor-272572/)

★ Diabetes Ratgeber & Dr. Sabine Haaß
(http://www.diabetes-ratgeber.net/Diabetes-Typ-1/Mit-Diabetes-in-Kindergarten-und-Schule-489671.html)

★ diaTribe
(http://diatribe.org/google-secures-patent-glucose-sensing-contact-lens)

- ★ Epoch Times & Sayer Ji
(http://www.theepochtimes.com/n3/815556-10-natural-substances-that-could-help-cure-type-1-diabetes/)
- ★ EuroStemCell
(http://www.eurostemcell.org/commentanalysis/making-insulin-producing-beta-cells-stem-cells-how-close-are-we)
- ★ Fool.com & Todd Campbell
(http://www.fool.com/investing/general/2014/04/27/can-marijuana-treat-diabetes.aspx)
- ★ Fox News
(http://www.foxnews.com/health/2014/07/16/study-one-injection-could-reverse-symptoms-type-2-diabetes.html)
- ★ Fox News & Loren Grush
(http://www.foxnews.com/health/2014/04/25/increasing-daily-coffee-consumption-may-protect-against-type-2-diabetes.html)
- ★ HealthLine.com & Allison Blass
(http://www.healthline.com/diabetesmine/is-there-a-conspiracy-preventing-a-diabetes-cure)
- ★ Integrity Applications
(http://www.integrity-app.com/the-glucotrack/the-products/)
- ★ LivBit.com
(http://www.livbit.com/article/2011/11/15/the-bluecircle-glucose-wristband-calculates-blood-sugar-as-you-workout/)
- ★ LiveScience
(http://www.livescience.com/49525-temporary-tattoos-blood-sugar-levels.html)
- ★ Live Strong
(http://www.LiveStrong.com)
- ★ Mayo Clinic
(http://www.mayoclinic.org/diseases-conditions/type-2-diabetes/diagnosis-treatment/treatment/txc-20169988)
- ★ Medical Express
(http://medicalxpress.com/news/2014-07-insulin-producing-cells-diabetes-video.html)
- ★ Medical Express & Enrique Rivero
(http://medicalxpress.com/news/2015-04-metformin-inexpensive-effective-underused-diabetics.html)
- ★ Medical News Today
(http://www.medicalnewstoday.com)
- ★ MedTronic
(http://www.medtronicdiabetes.com/products/continuous-glucose-monitoring)

- ★ Mirror & Andrew Gregory
(http://www.mirror.co.uk/news/uk-news/obesity-diabetes-risk-later-life-3095759
(http://www.mirror.co.uk/news/cure-diabetes-could-sight-scientists-3118865)

- ★ Mirror & Jonathan Symcox
(http://www.mirror.co.uk/news/uk-news/obesity-blood-test-doctors-could-3284765)

- ★ Mirror & Natalie Dickinson
(http://www.mirror.co.uk/lifestyle/health/red-wine-protects-against-diabetes-3038831)

- ★ National Review of Medicine & Owen Dyer
(http://www.nationalreviewofmedicine.com)

- ★ Science Alert
(http://www.sciencealert.com/scientists-have-made-a-temporary-tattoo-that-monitors-diabetics-glucose-levels-and-it-looks-awesome)

- ★ Science Daily & McGill University Health Centre
(https://www.sciencedaily.com/releases/2015/08/150813123428.htm)

- ★ Sky News
(http://news.sky.com/story/1629807/diabetes-cure-hope-after-cell-transplant-trial)

- ★ The Battalion & Zach Grinovich
(http://www.thebatt.com/science-technology/a-m-diabetes-research-could-end-painful-insulin-tests/article_758a325e-e70b-11e4-9e17-8347675638ce.html)

- ★ The Guardian & James Meikle
(http://www.theguardian.com/society/2015/apr/30/water-instead-of-sugary-drinks-cut-diabetes-2-risk-by-quarter)

- ★ The New York Times & Kasia Lipska
(http://www.nytimes.com/2014/04/26/opinion/sunday/the-global-diabetes-epidemic.html)

- ★ The Oregonian/OregonLive & Katy Muldoon
(http://www.oregonlive.com/health/index.ssf/2014/04/5_signs_you_should_get_tested.html)

- ★ TrendHunter.com
(http://www.trendhunter.com/trends/bluecircle-by-david-seo)

- ★ University of Lincoln
(http://www.lincoln.ac.uk/news/2016/04/1220.asp)

- ★ VisionAware.org
(http://www.visionaware.org/blog/visionaware-blog/googles-prototype-smart-contact-lens-measuring-blood-glucose-levels-for-people-with-diabetes-1418/12)

★ WSB-TV Atlanta
(http://www.wsbtv.com/news/local/medical-breakthrough-could-help-millions-diabetes-/53877314#__federated=1)

Finally I would like to say thank you for the following and often extremely informal images used in present book:

★ Blausen.com & WikiPedia
(Image credit: Pancreas)

★ David Seo
(Image credit: bluecircle)

★ Diabetes-Cure.me
(Image credit: Sugar Guard)

★ Google, Novartis & Alcon
(Image credit: Glucose-Sensing Contact Lens)

★ Integrity Applications
(Image credit: GlucoTrack DF-F)

★ Jacobs School of Engineering/UC San Diego
(Image credit: Diabetes Tattoo)

★ Library and Archives of Canada & WikiPedia
(Image credit: Dr. Frederick Banting, Charles H. Best)

★ Mannkind
(Image credit: Afrezza)

★ MediWise
(Image credit: GlucoWise)

★ MedTronic
(Image credit: MiniMed & Elite Sensor)

★ Mikael Häggström & WikiPedia
(Image credit: Main symptoms)

★ University of Toronto
(Image credit: Dr. Frederick Banting with Charles H. Best)

★ WikiPedia
(Image credit: Effect of insulin on glucose uptake and metabolism)

★ World Health Organization
(Image credit: Main complications)

Liability disclaimer

This book/e-book is not a substitute for medical and/or healthcare advice. Present book/e-book serves as the writer's interpretation of his personal Diabetes views, without specific advice on any personal requirements. Use of any information from this book or any other book or web site referred to is for general information only and does not represent advice either expressed or implied. You are encouraged to seek professional, medical or healthcare advice. Accordingly, the author, his publishers and affiliates disclaim that the information provided should not be treated as advice. Furthermore, it is a strict condition of the that any individual reading the book recognizes and accepts unreservedly that all information, analyses, projections, forecasts, expectations, or outcomes relating to past, present, or future medical treatments, pharmaceutical experiences, drugs, economic activity, or investment, are provided exclusively for academic purposes and that such information must not in any way be construed as general or personal advice. The author and/or publishers shall not be held liable for any losses or damages incurred by anyone who follows or acts on the opinions, views, or forecasts expressed in any form in this book/e-book, on any other websites or from individuals connected by hyperlink to or from this website.

Anyone reading this book is solely responsible for their interpretation of its contents and for their own decisions and actions. The foregoing applies also to correspondence *(including private emails)*, to posts on other websites *(including internet message boards and public discussion forums)*, and to articles published in other mass media. You should make your own enquiries before entering into any medical related, Diabetes related decision on the basis of the information or material on this book/e-book.

Please ensure you contact a doctor or a medical/healthcare adviser directly to discuss your particular circumstances and how the information provided applies to your situation. All readers should consult their own doctor, Diabetes advisor, healthcare advisor or other specialists before attempting to implement any of the contents discussed, and should always employ prudent policies and practices appropriate to their own particular/medical circumstances.

www.ingramcontent.com/pod-product-compliance
Lightning Source LLC
Chambersburg PA
CBHW071350280526
45787CB00001B/274
9781533116000